The Homeopathic Child

A Parent's Handbook To
Common Acute Ailments
Volume 1 (A-I)

LIZA CALACHE

Copyright © 2013 Liza Calache

All rights reserved.

ISBN: 1492947350
ISBN-13: 978-1492947356

DEDICATION

This book is dedicated to my beautiful baby girl, Grace-Kelly Jacqueline Fender. She is my miracle and reason for creating this book.

TABLE OF CONTENTS

ACCIDENTS/BROKEN BONES/BRUISES/CONCUSSIONS/FALLS/TRAUMAS 16
ALLERGIC REACTIONS 17
ALLERGIES 18
ASTHMA 21
BACKACHE MOTHER 25
BEDWETTING 36
BIRTHMARKS 33
BITES AND STINGS 34
BREATHING DIFFICULTIES BABY 35
BREASTFEEDING PROBLEMS 40
  MASTITIS 40
  ENGORGED BREASTS 42
  PAINFUL BREASTS 43
  MILK SUPPLY 45
  NIPPLE PROBLEMS 48
CARPAL TUNNEL SYNDROME 51
CHICKEN POX 53
CIRCUMCISION 56
COLIC 57
COMMON COLD 63
CONJUNCTIVITIS (PINK EYE) 74
CONSTIPATION 81
CONVULSIONS 88
COUGH 90
CRADLE CAP 107
DIAPER RASH 110
DIARRHEA 112
EARACHE 121
FEVER/FLU 128
HEATSTROKE 131
INSOMNIA 132

Disclaimer

This homeopathic materia medica and repertory set is provided for information purposes only, with no guarantee of accuracy. It is not intended as a substitute for medical advice, nor as a claim for the effectiveness of homeopathic remedies in treating any of the symptoms mentioned in these books. If the symptoms persist, seek professional medical advice. Minor symptoms can often be a sign of a more serious underlying condition.

About The Author

Liza Calache

Liza is a 3rd generation homeopath with formal education beginning at just 12 years old. Sitting amongst medical professionals, Liza took advantage of every learning opportunity presented to her. While studying under world-renowned homeopath and professor, Luc De Schepper, MD, Liza acquired a vast amount of knowledge that would set the stage for further homeopathic prospects. Upon completion of her formal education, which lasted 15 years, she began teaching and practicing alongside her mother, Martine Calache, CCH, DiHOM, RsHOM, FHom. While being able to practice and teach, Liza has also acquired a bachelor of science in Chemistry and was certified by the state of New Jersey as a secondary education teacher. She applied her knowledge of chemistry, homeopathy and education together and was able to write her own chemistry text book for high school students. During her time as a high school teacher, she was nominated for teacher of the year for her unique ability to work with disadvantaged students with low learning abilities and transform how they learn. In 2013, Liza was blessed with a baby girl that would change her life. Liza continues to teach and practice Homeopathy with her mother in the school they named, First Class Homeopathy.

Notes

Notes

INTRODUCTION

When you have a baby, the first thing you wish you had more of is probably time; time for yourself, time to sleep, time to take care of work/house. I'm sure I am not the first to tell you that babies are very demanding on your time, energy and resources. If you are not prepared for what to expect, it can really throw you for a loop. Many first time parents will say that they have experience either raising or helping to raise younger siblings or other family members or friends. However, when it's your own child, things are very different. The responsibility is 100% yours. Everything about that child you need to decide for them, including their healthcare choices, at least until they are old enough to decide for themselves anyway. Thankfully you have made the decision that homeopathy is going to be part of your child's healthcare choices. With these books, you will be shown how to bring relief to yours and your child's most common acute ailments. Usually a homeopath will consult several books to come to a conclusion for the correct remedy fitting the symptoms of the patient. The first kind of book is called a repertory where lists of symptoms are presented and all the remedies fitting those symptoms are listed. The next step is to narrow down the remedies to top two or three remedies by asking questions such as location, sensation and modalities (this will be further discussed in chapter 1). Once narrowed down, the next kind of book consulted is called a materia medica. This is a detail of each remedy and all the symptoms they present. The remedy chosen is the one that best fits the symptoms of the patient. However, with these books, all your answers are right here. These books are a repertory and materia medica of the most common ailments a child and their mother/caregiver will go through in their first few years of life as well as older children.

HOW TO USE THIS BOOK

These books are intended to be used as a quick and simple reference guide to finding the most appropriate homeopathic remedy based upon the symptoms of the child. It is a compilation of facts gathered from several well-known authors and trusted sources in homeopathy. Straight to the point, with all the facts you need to get the right remedy fast, and all in one book!

Homeopathy works by balancing the person's immune system so that it can heal itself of whatever ailment it is battling. Since homeopathy is a holistic form of alternative medicine, it is based on the symptoms of the whole body: mental, emotional and physical. To find the appropriate remedy, it is VITAL that ALL or AS MANY AS POSSIBLE symptoms are noted. The remedy that matches the symptoms is the best one to give. This is easier to do with an adult who can effectively communicate their symptoms to you. The challenge comes with a child and even more so with an infant who cannot speak yet. In these cases, the power of OBSERVATIONS becomes extremely useful. The key is to be as descriptive as possible with noting the symptoms. For example, your child might tell you, "My throat hurts." If I were to research "sore throat" in the books, I would find at least 50 remedies! Ask your child some questions to get a more descriptive answer. Here are some questions to help you out:

Where does it hurt? Is it your whole throat, or does one side hurt more than the other? Would it make it better if you drank some hot milk or any kind of hot beverage? Does it feel burning? Does it hurt when you swallow?

Obviously this becomes a challenge with an infant. So observe when the baby is eating, does she pull away from bottle or breast? Do they take little sips, pause, and resume? Are they scratching the outside of their throat?

Now that you have your description, it's time to look up the main symptom. Let's stick with sore throat as our example. Turn to page ____. When you find sore throat, you will see all the possible remedies for this ailment. Now that you have your description, all you have to do is match the remedy that most looks like your child's description. The first column tells you the name of the remedy with its common abbreviation. The second column tells you how that remedy is different from the other remedies in that section. You will find that there will be two or three remedies that could fit your description. In this case, the third column was added. The third column tells you how to distinguish that remedy from other close matches by listing the most common ailments that remedy has.

A Few Words About Potencies

Now that you have found the remedy you will give, what strength do you give the remedy and how do you give it? There are several ways to do this, but I will show you the most updated way that is absorbed into the body most efficiently. To do this it is important to understand what the different "potencies" or strengths are available and in which events they are most commonly used.

6C
30C
200C
1000C or 1M
10000C or 10M
100000C or 100M or CM

When you purchase a homeopathic remedy, on the tube should have the name of the remedy and a number and a letter after it. This number and letter indicate the potency or strength that the remedy was made in. Each potency has a different purpose. The rule of thumb in classical homeopathic prescribing is to take into account the persons sensitivity. We do not want make the person feel any worse than they already do. While homeopathy has no side-effects, it is possible to "aggravate" the persons symptoms. What this means is that you have chosen the correct remedy for their symptoms, but the potency was too strong for their immune system to handle. In this case, their symptoms are worsened until the aggravation wears off. In order to prevent aggravations, we do not want to give a potency that is too high. For children, it is best that 6C or 30C is given for everyday ailments such as cold, flu, teething, etc. When there is an emergency, the most common potencies used are 200C and 1M. Very rarely would anyone use 10M or CM potencies. As homeopaths, we always have two choices for potencies because of the sensitivities of the patient. If we know the person is sensitive, we start with the lower potency. If after giving we notice that it does not work, the next step is to increase the potency as it might have been too low. If again it does not work, it probably is safe to say you did not choose the correct remedy. How long do you wait to determine if you need to change potency or change remedy? Usually by 3-4 doses if there is no response, make the necessary changes.

Now that you know which potencies to use, how do you administer the remedy? As Hahnemann (founder of homeopathy) stated in his last edition of his manual (Organon of Homeopathy 6th edition), for acute situations the protocol is as follows:

2 pellets of the remedy in a 4 ounce bottle. Mix around. Take 1 teaspoon from bottle. Repeat as necessary until symptoms disappear. With each time the remedy is repeated, it is important to succus the bottle each time BEFORE you take it.

What are succussions?

A Succussion is a forceful hitting on the bottom of the bottle, usually with one's palm.

What is the purpose of succussions?

I try to explain this as simple as possible, and this is where some chemistry comes in. Every object contains energy. There are two main categories of energies that exist: kinetic and potential. Kinetic is energy of motion and potential is stored energy or energy of its position. If something is not moving or at rest, it has potential energy until it is in motion which will then change to kinetic energy. This is exactly what we want to do with the remedy. Each time we take the remedy, we want to "activate" the molecules and make sure they are "moving around" so we hit the bottom of the bottle; succussions. Each time the bottle is succussed, the remedy gets stronger. How is that possible? This is how the remedies were originally made when bought them in the little tubes. Homeopathic remedies are not made solely on dilutions.

How are homeopathic remedies made from the original substance?

One drop of the substance is needed and either 9 or 99 drops of alcohol is added. 9 drops to make an "X" potency, and 99 drops to make a "C" potency scale. For our purposes, we are using the "C" scale. So 99 drops of alcohol is added to the 1 drop of the plant extract, making it 100 drops…that's where the "C" comes from (from the latin for 100). If you were to stop here, this would just be a dilution…not a homeopathic remedy. To make it a remedy, it has been succussed 100 times. Now you will have a 1C remedy. To get to desired number, repeat the process. Thankfully, there is no need to make these remedies since there are several companies that have already done that for us. This information is useful if you were in the jungle and saw a plant of the remedy and decided to make a remedy there because you forgot your kit!

How many succussions do you do before you take the remedy?

You can do anywhere from 2-8 succussions but remember, this makes the remedy stronger each time it is done. Therefore, remember that the person's sensitivity is important here. We do not want to aggravate. If they are sensitive, a good rule is 2-4, if they are not they can probably handle 6-8.

ACCIDENTS/BROKEN/BRUISES
BONES/CONCUSSION/FALLS/TRAUMAS

These cases constitute medical emergencies and require immediate medical advice. Take these remedies on the way to the hospital. These remedies do not replace emergency medical care.

REMEDIES:

Arnica, Bellis Perennis, Bryonia, Hypericum, Ledum, Ruta, Symphytum

Remedy	Symptom Differentiation	Keynote Differentiation
Arn	Give immediately after trauma, concussion, accident, fall, bruise	This remedy has an affinity for the muscles, capillaries and cellular tissues. Contusions, stiffness, muscular pain, feel that bed is too hard, worse from slightest touch/jolt/movement/damp cold, better from lying with head lower than feet, #1 trauma remedy/accidents/falls/hemorrhaging, given to stop bleeding. If you have children, you will give this remedy to your child several times throughout their childhood. For falls and bleeding, give the highest potency you have.
Bell Per	Injury to breast	This remedy has an affinity for the muscles. Lameness, sprained feeling, good remedy after surgery, gout, worse from cold baths, boils, acne, varicose veins
Bry	Fractured ribs	Very thirsty especially if during a fever, sinuses are very dry (hint to remember: if dry think "bry"), pressure headaches

		that usually travel from forehead to occiput, or can start from left eye and move to the back of the head
Hyp	Nerve injury (especially to back, hands, and feet)	This remedy has an affinity for the nervous system, painful scars, worse after having tooth pulled
Led	Black and blue, black eye, hard object hit, wounds are cold to touch, worse with warmth	This remedy has an affinity for the joints and the skin. Rheumatism, poison-ivy-like rash, tetanus, twitching, better from cold, worse at night and from heat of bed
Ruta	Injury to knee, shin, elbow, periosteum, nodules	Dequervian syndrome, bone injuries, fractures with slow repair of broken bones, affinity for tendons, joints, wrists, ankles, cartilage, periosteum, and skin
Symph	Injury to cheekbone, bones around eyes, black and blue, speeds healing (if doesn't work, think of calc. phos)	

ALLERGIC REACTIONS

REMEDIES:

Apis

Remedy	Symptom Differentiation	Keynote Differentiation

Apis	Throat swelling, hives, puffy face, eyelids and under eyelids are swollen, cannot tolerate clothing or jewelry on neck, itchy body, worse night, skin feels swollen/tense/tight/sensitive to touch	This remedy is known for swelling, burning pain, and jealousy. Worse from heat, better from cold, hot dry skin, inflammation

ALLERGIES

REMEDIES:

Allium Cepa, Ambrosia, Arsenicum Album, Euphrasia, Kali Bich., Natrum Mur., Nux Vomica, Pulsatilla, Sabadilla, Sulphur, Wyethia

Remedy	Symptom Differentiation	Keynote Differentiation
All Cep	Nose discharge is profuse/watery/burning, worse damp and warm room, better from open air, eyes are red/tearing (non-irritating)/rubbing, nose feels raw and tingling, sneezing, headache	This remedy has an affinity for the upper respiratory mucus, intestines and nervous system. Cough is loud/raspy/spasmodic, worse in evening/heat/heated room, better in cool or open air, whooping cough
Amb	Hayfever, nose discharge is watery, eyes are itchy and tearing, throat is irritated, breathing is asthmatic	This remedy is known for hayfever symptoms, tearing and itching of eyes, diarrhea, worse during the symmer
Ars	Eyes are burning and tearing, worse on right side, better from	This remedy has an affinity for mucus, kidneys

	warm room, sneezes violently	liver, adrenal glands and the nervous system. This remedy can be summed up in three words: weak, restless and cold (temperature-wise). Burning pains, worse 1-3am and from the cold, thirsty for small amounts of cold water, fear of death, food-poisoning
Euph	Eyes are wartery/red/tearing, worse in open air/wind/lying down, nose discharge is non-irritating	This remedy has an affinity for the nose and the eyes. Pink eye, eyes clump together, worse heat/wind/night, better in the dark, measles
Kali Bich	Nose discharge is thick/gluey/stringy/yellow/post-nasal drip/sticky, sneezing	This remedy has an affinity for mucus and the skin. Worse cold/2-3am/movement/drinking beer, better with heat, pains start and stop suddenly, aphthae in mouth, thirsty for beer, burning pain in stomach, sciatica left side, heel pain, ulcers, headaches from digestive issues
Nat Mur	Hayfever attach in spring and fall, worse emotional trauma, sneezing, nose discharge profuse/watery/loss of taste/loss of smell/congestion,	This remedy can be summed up with three words: Malnutrition, dehydrated and weak. Worse being consoled,

	cold sores	worse 10am, worse when at the ocean, loss of vital fluids will cause symptoms, discharge is clear and in large quantities, craves salt, eczema in the creases of joints/forehead/edge of scalp, herpetic rashes especially after illness, dry and cracked skin, chapped lips
Nux Vom	Nose discharge in daytime only, congested at night, worse cold/uncovered/indoors, better in open air, sneezing, irritable, chilly	This remedy as an affinity for the nervous and digestive system. Irritable, cold, hypersensitive, angry, worse after eating, better with sleep, tongue is yellow/white color, craves spicy and sour food, constipation, sneezing upon waking
Puls	Nose discharge in daytime only, congested at night, worse in warm room/hot weather/lying down, better in open air/cool compresses/cool room, moody	This remedy has an affinity for the venous system and mucus. Changeable behavior, worse from heat, better from cold open air, thirstless, thick yellow/yellow-greenish discharge, worse after sunset
Sabad	Spasmodic sneezing, nose itchy and runny, eyes red and tearing,	This remedy has an affinity for the mucus of

	headache, lump in throat, desire to swallow, chilly, eyelids burning and red	the nose and tearing glands. Hayfever remedy, chilly, sore throat on the left side, better with warm drinks, thirstless,
Sul	Hayfever in summer, worse indoors, nose stuffy indoors/runny outdoors/red/discharge burns/smelly	This remedy has an affinity for the heart and skin. Worse standing still/heat of bed/water/11am, better perspiring/motion/dry weather, burning sensations all over body, eczema, craves sweets and open air, children look like they have a potbelly, children hate to take baths
Wye	Nose itchy (especially behind nose in roof of mouth), throat tickling/hacking cough/feels swollen/difficulty swallowing (even though constant desire to swallow)/dry	This remedy has an affinity for the throat. Irritable throat from singers and public speakers, hemorrhoids, hayfever

ASTHMA

REMEDIES:

Aconite, Antimonium Tart., Arsenicum Album, Chamomilla, Ipecacuanha, Lobelia, Nux Vomica, Pulsatilla, Sambucus, Spongia

Remedy	Symptom Differentiation	Keynote Differentiation

Acon	Beginning onset of asthmatic breathing, anxiety, fear, restlessness	This remedy has an affinity for the circulatory and nervous system. Worse extreme or sudden cold/extreme heat/night, better with perspiration, rapid pulse, sudden high fever, red skin, intense thirst for large quantities of cold water, restlessness, anxiety, fear of death, croup cough
Ant Tart	Cough is rattling, cannot bring up mucus, worse at 4am/anger/being annoyed/lying down, better sitting up, chilly	This remedy has an affinity for the respiratory system and the skin. This remedy can be summed up with three words: exhaustion, paleness, and sleepiness. Spitting behavior, grasps for other people
Ars	Breathing is better sitting straight up and warmth, worse from 12-2am and cold, restlessness, thirsty for small sips of water	This remedy has an affinity for mucus, kidneys liver, adrenal glands and the nervous system. This remedy can be summed up in three words: weak, restless and cold (temperature-wise).

		Burning pains, worse 1-3am and from the cold, thirsty for small amounts of cold water, fear of death, food-poisoning
Cham	Astham from tantrums, breathing is better bending head backwards/cold air/drinking cold water	This remedy has an affinity for the digestive system. Hypersensitive to pain, pain feels intolerable, numbness, irritable, angry, moody, hateful, exhausted from teething, insomnia, one cheek is red and hot while other is pale and cold, worse from anger/9pm and 12am/heat(toothache), better from being carried or riding in car
Ipecac	Wheezing, nausea, loose cough, rattling, vomiting, worse hot/humid weather/slightest motion, cold sweats, excessive saliva	This remedy has an affinity for the digestive and respiratory system. Hemorrhaging bright red blood, profuse saliva, not thirsty at all, disgusted by food, persistent and violent nausea, vomit is sticky and does not relieve nausea, stools are fermented like yeast, cough with suffocation,

		large amount of mucus
Lob	Asthma with nausea and vomiting, worse cold	Prickling sensation all over body, weakness in pit of stomach, lump feeling in sternum
Nux Vom	Asthma from full stomach, worse morning and after eating, choking, anxiety, noises in ear	This remedy as an affinity for the nervous and digestive system. Irritable, cold, hypersensitive, angry, worse after eating, better with sleep, tongue is yellow/white color, craves spicy and sour food, constipation, sneezing upon waking
Puls	Asthma from warm stuffy room and after eating fatty or rich foods	This remedy has an affinity for the venous system and mucus. Changeable behavior, worse from heat, better from cold open air, thirstless, thick yellow/yellow-greenish discharge, worse after sunset
Samb	Asthma during sleep (usually 3am), breathing is obstructed, worse from lying down/sleep/fruit, better from sitting up/motion/gasping for air, sweats profusely	This remedy has an affinity for the respiratory organs. Dry nose in infants, restlessness, colic, suffocative cough, choking cough (turns

		blue from cough)
Spon	Asthma with dry/barking/croupy cough, hoarseness, worse from cold air/warm room/tobacco/smoke/talking/lying with head low/drinking cold fluids/eating sweets/evening, better from warm food/warm drinks/sitting up/leaning forward	This remedy has an affinity of the respiratory mucus, glands, and lymphatic system. Worse at night/head lowered/inside hot room, better from hot drinks and raising head, dryness of nose and larynx

BACKACHE MOTHER REMEDIES:

Aesculus, Belladonna, Bryonia, Calcarea Carbonica, Calcarea Fluorica, Cimicifuga, Dulcamara, Ferrum Metallicum, Hypericum, Kali Carbonica, Kali Phos, Lycopodium, Mercurius Solibus, Natrum Muriaticum, Nux Vomica, Phosphorus, Pulsatilla, Rhododendrum, Rhus Tox, Sepia, Silica, Sulphur, Zinc

Remedy	Symptom Differentiation	Keynote Differentiation
Aesc	During pregnancy, worse standing up, worse rising from sitting position, lumbar pain localized in the sacro-iliac joints	Major hip remedy, generally better by creating better circulation such as exercise, cold, hemorrhoid remedy
Bell	Dragging down pain, During pregnancy, spasms, throbbing pain	Symptoms usually have sudden and violent onset, local congestion of blood (example face is red), the congested area is usually

		hot, children usually convulse when they have a fever
Bry	Lower back, stitching pain, piercing pain, searing pain, worse during cough, worse during menses, worse slightest movement, worse from heat, worse at night usually at 9pm, pain is better by rest, better with strong pressure,	Very thirsty especially if during a fever, sinuses are very dry (hint to remember: if dry think "bry"), pressure headaches that usually travel from forehead to occiput, or can start from left eye and move to the back of the head
Calc Carb	Lower back, aching pain, feels sprained, worse during damp weather, worse from cold, backache after lifting	Any Calcarea remedy has an affinity for bones, lymph nodes, circulation and polyps. They sweat profusely on head, babies teethe late, walk slow and are lazy, large appetite, remember the four F's: fat, fair skin, fainting, and fearful. If Ruta and Rhus Tox have stopped working, this remedy can be thought of. For chronic indications of pulsatilla
Calc Fluor	Lower back, better with continued movement, worse on beginning of motion, worse resting, better with heat and hot compresses	Any Calcarea remedy has an affinity for bones, lymph nodes, circulation and polyps. Teeth are irregularly arranged and small in size, and the enamel is poor quality. #1 remedy for bone spurs.

		Multiple sprains, Discharges are usually green or yellow. This remedy is for chronic indications of ruta and rhus tox
Cimi	Rheumatic pain, backache during pregnancy	
Dulc	Lower back, aching, sore and bruised pain, lameness, better with walking and movement, worse in wet weather, backache after change of weather, getting cold or wet	This remedy has an affinity for respiratory and digestive tract, lymphatic and muscular system, and the skin. Stuffy nose when exposed to cold, wet or rainy weather, catches a cold from air-conditioner, head cold in newborns
Ferr Met	Lower back, better walking slowly, worse on beginning of motion, dizziness when standing from lying position, worse washing in cold water	This remedy has an affinity for the blood and spleen. Mothers are never the same after childbirth. Pale and blush very easily. Weak, tired, sensitive to cold, cannot make effort, urinate involuntarily when coughing or sneezing or when children play, throbbing headache with hammering pain
Hyp	Coccyx pain, lower back pain, shooting pain, searing pain, sore and bruised pain, tearing pain, burning and tingling pain,	This remedy has an affinity for the nervous system, painful scars, worse after

	backache after childbirth, after epidural, after forceps delivery, after injury to coccyx or after injury to spine	having tooth pulled
Kali Carb	Lower back, dragging down pain, sore and bruised pain, stitching pain, shooting, burning and prickling pain, feels like they are stabbed with knife or needle, better lying on hard surface, better with pressure, worse specifically 3am time period, worse before menses, worse after sitting long period, worse walking, pains wander throughout the body, backache after posterior childbirth, backache after pregnancy	This remedy has an affinity for the nervous, digestive and respiratory system with specific action on lungs, mucus and blood. Weary, anemic and tired complexion, swelling inside upper eyelid, perspire easily, hypersensitive to noise and touch, anxiety, absent-minded, worse 2-5am, asthma which is better by sitting forward with elbows on knees, #1 stomach ulcer remedy, PMS remedy, flatulence
Kali Phos	Spine pain, sore and bruised feeling, better with motion and eating, better when in the company of pleasant friends/family	This remedy has an affinity for the nervous and muscular system as well as the blood. Weak, tired, and hypersensitive, worse over-nursing and over-stimulation of mind, discharges are golden, orange or bloody, irritable, moody, headaches in children, nightmares cause insomnia, vaginitis with brown discharge

Lyc	Lower back, stiffness, better with motion, better passing gas, better urinating, worse with beginning of motion, worse passing stool, worse getting up from sitting position, backache from lifting, burning pain between shoulder blades,	This remedy has an affinity for liver and digestion, kidneys and genitals, mucus and skin, and nervous system. Worse between 4-8pm, worse with heat, better with cool air, craving for sweets and oysters, ravenous appetite, flatulence, bloating after meals, doesn't like tight clothes on waist, abdomen is distended, red face after eating, migraine from poor digestion, bedwetting, nose stuffy with crusty mucus especially at night, sleep with mouth open, runny nose during day, anorexia in children
Merc Sol	Lower back, burning pain, shooting pain, worse breathing, worse coughing, worse sweating, worse getting up from sitting position, intolerance to slightest change in temperature	This remedy has an affinity for the digestive and renal systems with specific action on throat. Foul-smelling breath, gums are white/yellow color and ulcers in gums, tooth abscess, sores in mouth, intense thirst, thick tongue, salivate heavily, parotiditis, heavy perspiration especially at night and offensive in odor, ulcers, worse at night, known as "the human thermometer,"

		shivering and goose-bumps
Nat Mur	Lower back, aching pain, back feels broken, sore and bruised pain, better lying on hard surface, backache from physical labour	This remedy can be summed up with three words: Malnutrition, dehydrated and weak. Worse being consoled, worse 10am, worse when at the ocean, loss of vital fluids will cause symptoms, discharge is clear and in large quantities, craves salt, eczema in the creases of joints/forehead/edge of scalp, herpetic rashes especially after illness, dry and cracked skin, chapped lips,
Nat Sul	Sore and bruised pain, backache from injury to spine, better when changing position often, better passing heavy stool	This remedy has an affinity for digestive, respiratory and nervous system, with effects on the joints and skin, worse from cold and humidity, intense thirst especially for cold drinks, watery stool that squirt out especially in the morning, bronchitis, asthma in children, holds chest when coughing
Nux Vom	Lower back, aching pain, dragging down pain, pressing pain, worse sore and bruised pain, worse in the morning and worse with motion, backache	This remedy as an affinity for the nervous and digestive system. Irritable, cold, hypersensitive, angry, worse after eating, better

	from childbirth, getting cold and pregnancy	with sleep, tongue is yellow/white color, craves spicy and sour food, constipation, sneezing upon waking
Phos	Backache between shoulder blades, lower back, back feels broken, burning pain, better with rubbing, worse getting up from sitting position, backache from childbirth	This remedy is highly sensitive especially to light, noises, and smells. Fear of thunderstorm, worse from cold/storms/left side, better from sleep, craves salt and cold drinks, midnight "snacker" especially around 3 am, #1 morning sickness remedy
Puls	Lower back, small of back, dragging down pain, better with slow walking, worse with beginning of motion, worse before menses and during menses, worse getting up from sitting position, pains wander throughout body, backache from pregnancy	This remedy has an affinity for the venous system and mucus. Changeable behavior, worse from heat, better from cold open air, thirstless, thick yellow/yellow-greenish discharge, worse after sunset
Rhod	Neck pain, lower back pain, sore and bruised pain, searing pain, better with motion, worse with wet weather, worse right before a storm, better after the storm has passed	This remedy has an affinity for the muscular system.
Rhus Tox	Neck pain, lower back pain, aching pain, dragging down pain, sore and bruised pain, stiffness,	This remedy has an affinity for the skin, mucus and the nervous system. Better

		better lying on hard surface, better with motion, better walking, worse with beginning of motion, worse reaching up motion, worse getting up from sitting position, worse wet weather, backache from damp weather, backache from injury, backache from lifting, sciatica with tearing pains, pains shoot along the nerve, backache from pregnancy, bachache from sprain	with slow motion and changing of position, shivers when slights part of body is uncovered, perspiration all over body except the face, sprains and dislocations, worse 4-5am and 7pm, intense thirst for cold water or milk
	Sep	Lower back, aching pain, dragging down pain, tugging pain in back and sacrum, better with pressure, worse bending down, worse afternoon time, worse before and during menses, worse night, worse sitting position	This remedy has an affinity for the circulatory and nervous system. Hormonal imbalance. Sitting or kneeling for long periods causes fainting, worse before storm, better with exercise, feels like abdomen is heavy, flushes of heat in face, craves vinegar, and sour foods, worse 11 am,
	Sil	Sore and bruised pain, stitching pain, stiffness, lameness, worse during breastfeeding, worse at night, worse with pressure, worse sitting position, worse getting up from sitting position, backache from fall on back, backache from physical labour	This remedy has an affinity for the nervous system and is very malnourished. They are weak and demineralized. Worse cold and humid weather, better with heat, slinters (will push them out), fontanels stay open, perspire on head, abscess remedy, white spots on nails, weak nails/hair

Sul	Lower back, aching pain, sore and bruised pain, burning pain, throbbing pain, stiffness, weakness, worse bending down motion, worse during menses, worse at night, worse after sitting long period of time, worse walking	This remedy has an affinity for the heart and skin. Worse standing still/heat of bed/water/11am, better perspiring/motion/dry weather, burning sensations all over body, eczema, craves sweets and open air, children look like they have a potbelly, children hate to take baths
Zinc	Coccyx pain, neck pain, spine pain, aching pain, sore and bruised pain, weakness, worse sitting position, worse writing,	Restless leg syndrome, worse alcohol especially wine, better with any discharge

BIRTHMARKS

REMEDIES:

Remedy	Symptom Differentiation	Keynote Differentiation
Thuja		This remedy has an affinity for the skin, mucus, and any type of growths appearing inside of body or outside on the skin: warts, moles, acne, seborrhea, cradle cap, hair loss, scalp has white scaly dandruff Worse cold/humid weather/3 am or 3 pm, better with heat, discharges have a

		moldy smell

BITES AND STINGS

REMEDIES:

Apis, Hypericum, Ledum, Staphysagria

Remedy	Symptoms Differentiation	Keynote Differentiation
Apis	Bite is red and inflamed, burning and stitching pain, worse from heat or warm compresses, better from cold or cold compresses	This remedy is known for swelling, burning pain, and jealousy. Worse from heat, better from cold, hot dry skin, inflammation
Hyp	Bite pain is sharp and shooting	This remedy has an affinity for the nervous system, painful scars, worse after having tooth pulled
Led	Bite is itching and stinging, better from cold compresses	This remedy has an affinity for the joints and the skin. Rheumatism, poison-ivy-like rash, tetanus, twitching, better from cold, worse at night and from heat of bed
Staph	Bite is excessively itchy, welts	This remedy has an affinity for the urinary and genital system as well as the skin. Hypersensitive to emotions, excitable, irritated easily, obsessed about sexual ideas, burning/frequent/dripping urination, eczema with severe

		itching, styes especially on upper eyelids

BITING

REMEDIES:

Remedy	Symptom Differentiation	Keynote Differentiation
Bell		Symptoms usually have sudden and violent onset, local congestion of blood (example face is red), the congested area is usually hot, children usually convulse when they have a fever

BREATHING PROBLEMS IN NEWBORN

REMEDIES:

Antimonium Tart., Carbo Veg.

Remedy	Symptom Differentiation	Keynote Differentiation
Ant Tart	Rattling of mucus, shortness of breath, frequent respiration when lying down, grasps larynx when coughing, breathing is noisy, expectoration is very difficult	This remedy has an affinity for the respiratory system and the skin. This remedy can be summed up with three words: exhaustion, paleness, and sleepiness. Spitting behavior, grasps

		for other people
Carbo Veg	Desires to be fanned, burping, cyanosis, asphyxia in newborns, excessive perspiration, faint-like feeling	This remedy has an affinity for the digestive system and the body's circulation. Lack of reaction, engorged veins, slow recovery of previous illness, sluggish, listless, indifferent

BEDWETTING

REMEDIES:

Belladonna, Carbo Veg., Causticum, Equisetum, Ferrum Phos, Kreosotum, Lycopodium, Phosphoricum Acid., Pulsatilla, Sepia, Sulphur

Remedy	Symptom Differentiation	Keynote Differentiation
Bell		Symptoms usually have sudden and violent onset, local congestion of blood (example face is red), the congested area is usually hot, children usually convulse when they have a fever
Carbo Veg	Bedwetting during first stage of sleep and/or early morning	This remedy has an affinity for the digestive system and the body's circulation. Lack of reaction, engorged veins, slow recovery of previous illness, sluggish,

		listless, indifferent
Caust	Worse winter, better summer, fears something bad will happen, fears the dark, involuntary urination on sneezing or coughing, feeling like the bladder is paralyzed	This remedy can be summed up in two words: weakness and paralysis. Worse cold/3-4am/when thinking about symptoms, better with heat and humidity and cold water, warts under the nails, crave smoked foods
Equis	Bedwetting out of habit, nightmares, wild dreams during bedwetting, dreams of crowds of people	This remedy has an affinity for the urinary mucosa. Kidney regulator.
Ferr Phos	Bedwetting during daytime, feels urge to urinate while standing, better lying down	Tired, anemic, pale. Bleeds easily, low temperature, rapid pulse, face is red and pale alternatingly, hemorrhages easily, better with slow motion, craves sour things
Kreos	Sudden urge to urinate while in bed not having enough time to get up, bedwetting during first stage of sleep, dreams of urinating	This remedy has an affinity for mucus and tends to hemorrhage.
Lyc	Worries about what others will think of him, bedwetting worse in warm or stuffy room, sleeps with window open	This remedy has an affinity for liver and digestion, kidneys and genitals, mucus and skin, and nervous system. Worse between 4-8pm, worse with heat,

		better with cool air, craving for sweets and oysters, ravenous appetite, flatulence, bloating after meals, doesn't like tight clothes on waist, abdomen is distended, red face after eating, migraine from poor digestion, bedwetting, nose stuffy with crusty mucus especially at night, sleep with mouth open, runny nose during day, anorexia in children, fear of new things, "devil at home and angel outside syndrome", lack of self-confidence
Phos Ac	Loss of control of organs/limbs	This remedy is severely exhausted especially because of emotional upset. Symptoms are caused by a loss of fluids, indifference to everything, fatigue, painless and orderless diarrhea, urine is milky colored, urine can also be clear in color, hair loss all over body
Puls	Urge to urinate when lying flat on back, bedwetting before and during measles.	This remedy has an affinity for the venous system and mucus. Changeable behavior, worse from heat, better from cold open air, thirstless, thick

			yellow/yellow-greenish discharge, worse after sunset, sleeps with feet uncovered
	Sep	Bedwetting right after falling asleep and/or early evening before 10pm	This remedy has an affinity for the circulatory and nervous system. Hormonal imbalance. Sitting or kneeling for long periods causes fainting, worse before storm, better with exercise, feels like abdomen is heavy, flushes of heat in face, craves vinegar, and sour foods, worse 11 am
	Sul		This remedy has an affinity for the heart and skin. Worse standing still/heat of bed/water/11am, better perspiring/motion/dry weather, burning sensations all over body, eczema, craves sweets and open air, children look like they have a potbelly, children hate to take baths, wakes at 5am, vivid dreams, sleeps with feet uncovered

BREASTFEEDING PROBLEMS

MASTITIS

REMEDIES:

Hepar Sulphur, Mercurius Sol, Phytolaca, Silica, Sulphur

Remedy	Symptom Differentiation	Keynote Differentiation
Hep Sul	Inflamed breasts, skin looks unhealthy, skin is sensitive to touch	This remedy is hypersensitive especially to touch and cold air, worse dry/cold weather/slightest draft, better with heat, craves sour things especially vinegar
Merc Sol	Painful breasts	This remedy has an affinity for the digestive and renal systems with specific action on throat. Foul-smelling breath, gums are white/yellow color and ulcers in gums, tooth abscess, sores in mouth, intense thirst, thick tongue, salivate heavily, parotiditis, heavy perspiration especially at night and offensive in odor, ulcers, worse at night, known as "the human thermometer," shivering and goose-bumps
Phyt	Inflamed breasts, painful while nursing, painful before and during menses, hard,	This remedy has an affinity for the mucus, breasts and bones. Worse with

		woody and painful nodules, cracked nipples	cold/wet/motion, better with dry weather and resting. Stiffness and bruising all over body, sciatica
	Sil	Inflamed breasts, painful, painful while nursing, cutting and stitching pain, pain is worse on left side	This remedy has an affinity for the nervous system and is very malnourished. They are weak and demineralized. Worse cold and humid weather, better with heat, slinters (will push them out), fontanels stay open, perspire on head, abscess remedy, white spots on nails, weak nails/hair
	Sul	Inflamed breasts, and red	This remedy has an affinity for the heart and skin. Worse standing still/heat of bed/water/11am, better perspiring/motion/dry weather, burning sensations all over body, eczema, craves sweets and open air, children look like they have a potbelly, children hate to take baths

ENGORGED BREASTS

REMEDIES:

Belladonna, Bryonia

Remedy	Symptom Differentiation	Keynote Differentiation
Bell	Hard, hot, inflamed breasts, painful, throbbing pain, red-streaked	Symptoms usually have sudden and violent onset, local congestion of blood (example face is red), the congested area is usually hot, children usually convulse when they have a fever
Bry	Hard, hot, inflamed breasts, painful, pain is worse with the slightest movement	Very thirsty especially if during a fever, sinuses are very dry (hint to remember: if dry think "bry"), pressure headaches that usually travel from forehead to occiput, or can start from left eye and move to the back of the head

PAIN IN BREASTS

REMEDIES:

Belladonna, Borax, Bryonia, Mercurius Sol, Sepia, Silica

Remedy	Symptom Differentiation	Keynote Differentiation
Bell	Throbbing pain, red-streaked	Symptoms usually have sudden and violent onset, local congestion of blood (example face is red), the congested area is usually hot, children usually convulse when they have a fever
Bor	Aching pain after nursing	This remedy has an affinity for the nervous system, skin and mucus of the mouth. Thrush, aphthae of mouth, refuse to eat because painful patches inside cheeks, skin looks unhealthy, worse leaning forward/downward/falling motion
Bry	Slightest movement makes pain worse	Very thirsty especially if during a fever, sinuses are very dry (hint to remember: if dry think "bry"), pressure headaches that usually travel from forehead to occiput, or can start from left eye and move to the back of the head
Merc Sol		This remedy has an affinity for the digestive and renal

		systems with specific action on throat. Foul-smelling breath, gums are white/yellow color and ulcers in gums, tooth abscess, sores in mouth, intense thirst, thick tongue, salivate heavily, parotiditis, heavy perspiration especially at night and offensive in odor, ulcers, worse at night, known as "the human thermometer," shivering and goose-bumps
Sep		This remedy has an affinity for the circulatory and nervous system. Hormonal imbalance. Sitting or kneeling for long periods causes fainting, worse before storm, better with exercise, feels like abdomen is heavy, flushes of heat in face, craves vinegar, and sour foods, worse 11 am
Sil	Pain while nursing, cutting/stitching pain, worse left breast while nursing	This remedy has an affinity for the nervous system and is very malnourished. They are weak and demineralized. Worse cold and humid weather, better with heat, slinters (will push them out), fontanels stay open, perspire on head, abscess remedy, white spots on nails, weak

		nails/hair

MILK SUPPLY

REMEDIES:

Belladonna, Bryonia, Calcarea Carb., Caustium, Dulcamara, Lac Defloratum, Pulsatilla, Secale, Urtica Urens, Lac Cininum

Remedy	Symptom Differentiation	Keynote Differentiation
Bell	Over-abundant supply	Symptoms usually have sudden and violent onset, local congestion of blood (example face is red), the congested area is usually hot, children usually convulse when they have a fever
Bry	Over-abundant supply	Very thirsty especially if during a fever, sinuses are very dry (hint to remember: if dry think "bry"), pressure headaches that usually travel from forehead to occiput, or can start from left eye and move to the back of the head
Calc Carb	Low/Over-abundant supply	Any Calcarea remedy has an affinity for bones, lymph nodes, circulation and polyps.

		They sweat profusely on head, babies teethe late, walk slow and are lazy, large appetite, remember the four F's: fat, fair skin, fainting, and fearful. If Ruta and Rhus Tox have stopped working, this remedy can be thought of. For chronic indications of pulsatilla
Caust	Low supply	This remedy can be summed up in two words: weakness and paralysis. Worse cold/3-4am/when thinking about symptoms, better with heat and humidity and cold water, warts under the nails, crave smoked foods
Dulc	Low supply, in chilly women	This remedy has an affinity for respiratory and digestive tract, lymphatic and muscular system, and the skin. Stuffy nose when exposed to cold, wet or rainy weather, catches a cold from air-conditioner, head cold in newborns

Lac C	To end milk supply	This remedy has an affinity for the breasts. Painful swelling of breasts, better with beginning menses, dreams of snakes
Lac D	Low supply	This remedy has an affinity for the body's nutrition. Diarrhea in infants, body smells sour, headache with intense throbbing pain in forehead, constipation, indigestion, doesn't want milk, worse after drinking milk, thick white urine
Puls	Over-abundant supply, To end milk supply	This remedy has an affinity for the venous system and mucus. Changeable behavior, worse from heat, better from cold open air, thirstless, thick yellow/yellow-greenish discharge, worse after sunset
Sec	Low supply	This remedy has an affinity for the arterial walls and the uterus. Worse heat, better cold, burning sensations even though area may be cold

		to touch, body is cold and does not want to be covered, violent cramping especially in legs, hemorrhaging (black blood)
Urt U	Low/Over-abundant supply	This remedy has an affinity for the skin. Burning, pricking pains and swelling, worse with cold compresses, hives from eating seafood, gout

NIPPLE PROBLEMS

REMEDIES:

Castor Equi, Causticum, Phytolacca, Sarsparilla, Sepia, Silica, Sulphur

Remedy	Symptom Differentiation	Keynote Differentiation
Castor	Cracked and ulcerated nipples, sore, swollen, tender to touch, violent itching, red areola, warts on breasts	This remedy has an affinity for the skin, female organs, nails, and bones. Warts on forehead and breast, pain coccyx
Caust	Cracked, sore	This remedy can be summed up in two words: weakness and paralysis. Worse cold/3-4am/when thinking about symptoms, better with heat and humidity and cold water,

			warts under the nails, crave smoked foods
	Phyt	Cracked, sore, pain during nursing	This remedy has an affinity for the mucus, breasts and bones. Worse with cold/wet/motion, better with dry weather and resting. Stiffness and bruising all over body, sciatica
	Sars	Cracked, sore, itching	This remedy has an affinity for the skin and mucus. Dry/shriveled/creased skin, purple and blue spots on skin, pain after urinating, unable to urinate while sitting-must stand, intense pain in kidneys especially right kidney
	Sep	Cracked, sore, bleeding, inverted, retracted	This remedy has an affinity for the circulatory and nervous system. Hormonal imbalance. Sitting or kneeling for long periods causes fainting, worse before storm, better with exercise, feels like abdomen is heavy, flushes of heat in face, craves vinegar, and sour foods, worse 11 am
	Sil	Inverted, retracted nipples	This remedy has an affinity for the nervous system and is very malnourished. They

		are weak and demineralized. Worse cold and humid weather, better with heat, slinters (will push them out), fontanels stay open, perspire on head, abscess remedy, white spots on nails, weak nails/hair
Sul	Cracked, sore, itching	This remedy has an affinity for the heart and skin. Worse standing still/heat of bed/water/11am, better perspiring/motion/dry weather, burning sensations all over body, eczema, craves sweets and open air, children look like they have a potbelly, children hate to take baths

BURNS

REMEDIES:

Calendula, Cantharis, Causticum

Remedy	Symptom Differentiation	Keynote Differentiation
Calen	1st remedy to consider for burns, stops infection, first degree burns	Healing of wounds

Canth	Second and third degree burns, sunburns	This remedy has an affinity for the urinary tract and the skin. Pain is sharp (causes crying)/violent/piercing/burning in bladder, tendency to gangrene, feel like being "roasted alive" (intensity of burning pain), cystitis
Caust	First degree burns, speeds up healing	This remedy can be summed up in two words: weakness and paralysis. Worse cold/3-4am/when thinking about symptoms, better with heat and humidity and cold water, warts under the nails, crave smoked foods

CARPAL TUNNEL SYNDROME

REMEDIES:

Calcarea Phos., Causticum, Guaiacum, Hypericum, Ruta, Viola Odorata

Remedy	Symptom Differentiation	Keynote Differentiation
Calc Phos	Pain in bones and nerves of wrist and arms, stiffness and discomfort, cold weather and draft air makes discomfort worse	This remedy has an affinity for the bones, blood, lymph nodes and works on the nutrition of the body. Teeth are long, narrow and yellow, bones are long and straight, tired and nervous, rickets, weight loss, repetitive sore

		throat/bronchitis/colds
Caust	Bruised feeling, drawing, burning pain, stiffness, weakness, feels contractions of muscles in hands and forearm, worse cold, better warm, better rainy weather	This remedy can be summed up in two words: weakness and paralysis. Worse cold/3-4am/when thinking about symptoms, better with heat and humidity and cold water, warts under the nails, crave smoked foods
Guai	Stiff, burning pain, better icy cold application, tightness, feels need to stretch wrist	Tendons are too short, muscular pain, stitching pain, drawing pain, tense pain, swollen joints, worse heat, better cold, gout, abscess of joints, tonsilitis,
Hyp	Sharp, shooting pain extending to wrist	This remedy has an affinity for the nervous system, painful scars, worse after having tooth pulled , Nerve injury, Nervous conditions
Ruta	Overuse of joints, irritation of nerves, stiffness, bruised, lame feeling, weakness	Dequervian syndrome, bone injuries, fractures with slow repair of broken bones, affinity for tendons, joints, wrists, ankles, cartilage, periosteum, and skin
Viola	Right-sided, pain, numbness extends from wrist through hand to	Quarrelsome, easily offended, disobedient, restless

	fingers, arms tremble	

CHICKENPOX

REMEDIES:

Aconite, Antimonium Crudum, Antimonium Tart., Apis Belladonna, Mercurius Sol., Pulsatilla, Rhus Tox, Sulphur

Remedy	Symptom Differentiation	Keynote Differentiation
Acon	First stageart, chickenpox with fever	This remedy has an affinity for the circulatory and nervous system. Worse extreme or sudden cold/extreme heat/night, better with perspiration, rapid pulse, sudden high fever, red skin, intense thirst for large quantities of cold water, restlessness, anxiety, fear of death, croup cough
Ant Crud	Chickenpox with cough	This remedy has an affinity for the digestive tract, especially the stomach, and the skin. Tongue has thick white coating, thrush, burping, watery diarrhea, impetigo, warts, thick and hard nails, worse cold bath/radiating heat/over-eating

Ant Tart	Chickenpox with cough, rash is slowly appearing, chickenpox with respiratory problems	This remedy has an affinity for the respiratory system and the skin. This remedy can be summed up with three words: exhaustion, paleness, and sleepiness. Spitting behavior, grasps for other people
Apis	Chickenpox is itching and stinging, worse in warm room, better from cold and in cold room	This remedy is known for swelling, burning pain, and jealousy. Worse from heat, better from cold, hot dry skin, inflammation
Bell	Chickenpox with fever and with headache	Symptoms usually have sudden and violent onset, local congestion of blood (example face is red), the congested area is usually hot, children usually convulse when they have a fever
Merc Sol	Chickenpox with pus formations	This remedy has an affinity for the digestive and renal systems with specific action on throat. Foul-smelling breath, gums are white/yellow color and ulcers in gums, tooth abscess, sores in mouth, intense thirst, thick tongue, salivate heavily, parotiditis, heavy perspiration especially at night and offensive in odor, ulcers,

		worse at night, known as "the human thermometer," shivering and goose-bumps
Puls	Chickenpox with cough	This remedy has an affinity for the venous system and mucus. Changeable behavior, worse from heat, better from cold open air, thirstless, thick yellow/yellow-greenish discharge, worse after sunset, sleeps with feet uncovered
Rhus Tox	Chickenpox with rash itching violently	This remedy has an affinity for the skin, mucus and the nervous system. Better with slow motion and changing of position, shivers when slights part of body is uncovered, perspiration all over body except the face, sprains and dislocations, worse 4-5am and 7pm, intense thirst for cold water or milk
Sul	Chickenpox with rash itching violently	This remedy has an affinity for the heart and skin. Worse standing still/heat of bed/water/11am, better perspiring/motion/dry weather, burning sensations all over body, eczema, craves sweets and open air, children look like they have

		a potbelly, children hate to take baths, wakes at 5am, vivid dreams, sleeps with feet uncovered

CIRCUMCISION

REMEDIES:

Arnica, Calendula, Staphysagria

Remedy	Symptom Differentiation	Keynote Differentiation
Arn	To reduce shock before and after procedure	AetThis remedy has an affinity for the muscles, capillaries and cellular tissues. Contusions, stiffness, muscular pain, feel that bed is too hard, worse from slightest touch/jolt/movement/damp cold, better from lying with head lower than feet, #1 trauma remedy/accidents/falls/hemorrhaging, given to stop bleeding. If you have children, you will give this remedy to your child several times throughout their childhood. For falls and bleeding, give the highest potency you have.
Calen	Anti-septic	Healing of wounds
Staph	Wounds due to surgery	This remedy has an affinity for the urinary and genital system as well as the skin. Hypersensitive to emotions, excitable, irritated easily, obsessed about sexual ideas,

		burning/frequent/dripping urination, eczema with severe itching, styes especially on upper eyelids

COLIC

REMEDIES:

Aethusa, Allium Cepa, Belladonna, Chamomilla, Colocynthis, Cuprum Metallicum, Dioscorea, Ipecacuanha, Lycopodium, Magnesium Mur., Mangnesium Phos., Natrum Phos., Natrum Sulph., Nux Vomica, Secale, Staphysagria

Remedy	Symptom Differentiation	Keynote Differentiation
Aeth	Unable to digest mother's milk, regurgitates milk, sweating, weakness, restlessness, anxiety, crying	This remedy has an affinity for the digestive and nervous system. Profuse diarrhea and severe vomiting, cannot tolerate milk, total exhaustion, no thirst, consequences of over-feeding child, lack of concentration in children
All Cep	Colic and common cold	This remedy has an affinity for the upper respiratory mucus, intestines and nervous system. Cough is loud/raspy/spasmodic, worse in evening/heat/heated room, better in cool or open air, whooping cough

Bell	Spasms appear and disappear suddenly	Symptoms usually have sudden and violent onset, local congestion of blood (example face is red), the congested area is usually hot, children usually convulse when they have a fever
Cham	Colic in newborn, stomach/abdomen feels bloated, colic with diarrhea, angry disposition when "colicky"	This remedy has an affinity for the digestive system. Hypersensitive to pain, pain feels intolerable, numbness, irritable, angry, moody, hateful, exhausted from teething, insomnia, one cheek is red and hot while other is pale and cold, worse from anger/9pm and 12am/heat(toothache), better from being carried or riding in car
Coloc	Colic in newborns, stomach/abdomen feels bloated, cutting/griping/tearing/violent pain, pain comes in waves, colic with diarrhea/nausea/vomiting, worse after drinking/cold drinks/fruit/before stool, better passing stool and pressure, angry disposition when "colicky," colic from excitement/fruit/suppressed anger	This remedy has an affinity for the digestive and nervous system. Violent pain causing screaming, cramping pain comes suddenly, worse from anger/rest/left side, better from strong pressure, heat, bending forward, movement, painful diarrhea, facial neuralgia, sciatica

Cup	Cramping and violent pain, nausea and vomiting, hiccups, makes loud noises when swallowing	This remedy has an affinity for the muscular system. Spasmodic pain begins and ends suddenly, convulsions, blue face, violent cramping, whooping cough, better drinking a sip of cold water, violent diarrhea with cramping pains
Dios	Colic in newborns, abdomen/stomach is rumbling and gassy, pain in and around belly button, cutting/griping/twisting pain, worse bending forward and in the morning, better bending backward and stretching out	This remedy is mainly a colic remedy. Worse bending forward, better standing straight and bending backwards
Ipec	Aching/cramping/griping pain, worse with movement	This remedy has an affinity for the digestive and respiratory system. Hemorrhaging bright red blood, profuse saliva, not thirsty at all, disgusted by food, persistent and violent nausea, vomit is sticky and does not relieve nausea, stools are fermented like yeast, cough with suffocation, large amount of mucus
Lyc	Gassy, worse 4-8pm	This remedy has an affinity for liver and digestion, kidneys and genitals, mucus

			and skin, and nervous system. Worse between 4-8pm, worse with heat, better with cool air, craving for sweets and oysters, ravenous appetite, flatulence, bloating after meals, doesn't like tight clothes on waist, abdomen is distended, red face after eating, migraine from poor digestion, bedwetting, nose stuffy with crusty mucus especially at night, sleep with mouth open, runny nose during day, anorexia in children, fear of new things, "devil at home and angel outside syndrome", lack of self-confidence
Mag Mur		Colic in newborns, cramping/sore/bruised pain, colic with constipation/diarrhea/indigestion, worse after drinking milk, colic from teething	This remedy has an affinity for the digestive and uterine system. Worse from salt (eating and being by sea) and drinking milk, better by pressure, tongue has teeth marks, constipation with hard stools like that of sheep droppings, migraines better with wrapping heat with warm compress
Mag Phos		Cramping and drawing pain, better bending completely	This remedy has an affinity for the muscular system. It

		over/warmth/pressure	is a spasmodic remedy. Sudden/intolerable/cramping pains, worse from cold and right side, better from heat and leaning forward
Nat Phos		Abdomen/stomach feels bloated, colic with diarrhea and sour smelling vomit, gas smells sour, colic with worms	This remedy has an affinity for the digestive system. Worse eating sugar, inflammation in throat, lump feeling in throat, inside mouth and on tongue has thick yellow coating gas, jaundice, weakness,
Nat Sulph		Colic with indigestion	This remedy has an affinity for digestive, respiratory and nervous system, with effects on the joints and skin, worse from cold and humidity, intense thirst especially for cold drinks, watery stool that squirt out especially in the morning, bronchitis, asthma in children, holds chest when coughing
Nux Vom		Cramping and pressing pain, worse after eating/coughing/fever/morning/tight clothes, better with hot drinks/warmth of bed/passing gas/passing stool	This remedy as an affinity for the nervous and digestive system. Irritable, cold, hypersensitive, angry, worse after eating, better with sleep, tongue is yellow/white color, craves spicy and sour food,

			constipation, sneezing upon waking
	Sec	Colic in newborns, abdomen/stomach feels bloated, colic with diarrhea, colic from oxytocin drug intake	This remedy has an affinity for the arterial walls and the uterus. Worse heat, better cold, burning sensations even though area may be cold to touch, body is cold and does not want to be covered, violent cramping especially in legs, hemorrhaging (black blood)
	Staph	Cramping pain, worse after drinking, colic from being humiliated and suppressed anger	This remedy has an affinity for the urinary and genital system as well as the skin. Hypersensitive to emotions, excitable, irritated easily, obsessed about sexual ideas, burning/frequent/dripping urination, eczema with severe itching, styes especially on upper eyelids

COMMON COLD

REMEDIES:

Aconite, Allium Cepa, Arsenicum Album, Baryta Carb., Belladonna, Bryonia, Calcarea Carb., Calcarea Fluor., Calcarea Phos., Calcarea Sulph., Carbo Veg., Dulcamara, Euphrasia, Hepar Sulph., Kali Bich., Kali Mur., Kali Sulph., Lycopodium, Magnesia Mur., Mercurius Sol., Natrum Carb., Natrum Mur., Nitric Acid., Nux Vomica, Phosphoricum Acid., Phosphorus, Pulsatilla, Sepia, Silica, Sulphur

Remedy	Symptom Differentiation	Keynote Differentiation
Acon	Cold from getting chilled/cold/dry wind/shock	This remedy has an affinity for the circulatory and nervous system. Worse extreme or sudden cold/extreme heat/night, better with perspiration, rapid pulse, sudden high fever, red skin, intense thirst for large quantities of cold water, restlessness, anxiety, fear of death, croup cough
All Cep	Eyes streaming/non-irritating/watery discharge, nose discharge burns/profuse/from one side/watery/streaming, sneezing, nose discharge drips so much it burns the upper lip area around the nostrils, cold with headache, sore throat, worse in	This remedy has an affinity for the upper respiratory mucus, intestines and nervous system. Cough is loud/raspy/spasmodic, worse in

	stuffy room, better fresh air, cold from cold wind and getting wet feet	evening/heat/heated room, better in cool or open air, whooping cough
Ars	Eyes dry and burning, eyelids are red and puffy, nose discharge is burning/profuse/watery, sinuses are blocked and painful, sneezing, worse evening and the right side, cold from getting chilled	This remedy has an affinity for mucus, kidneys liver, adrenal glands and the nervous system. This remedy can be summed up in three words: weak, restless and cold (temperature-wise). Burning pains, worse 1-3am and from the cold, thirsty for small amounts of cold water, fear of death, food-poisoning
Bary C	Glands swollen, nose is dry, coughing, worse at night	This remedy has an affinity for the mental development, arteries, and lymphatic system. Late development/milestones, shy, worse cold/humid/thinking about problems
Bell	Cold with headache, fever, loss of taste and smell, cold from getting chilled/cold/dry wind/wet head	Symptoms usually have sudden and violent onset, local congestion of blood (example face is red), the congested area is usually hot,

		children usually convulse when they have a fever
Bry	Cold with headache, sneezing	Very thirsty especially if during a fever, sinuses are very dry (hint to remember: if dry think "bry"), pressure headaches that usually travel from forehead to occiput, or can start from left eye and move to the back of the head
Calc Carb	Dry/stuffy nose/congestion without discharge, if there is discharge from nose, it is smelly and yellow, painless hoarseness, loss of smell, worse in morning	Any Calcarea remedy has an affinity for bones, lymph nodes, circulation and polyps. They sweat profusely on head, babies teethe late, walk slow and are lazy, large appetite, remember the four F's: fat, fair skin, fainting, and fearful. If Ruta and Rhus Tox have stopped working, this remedy can be thought of
Calc Fluor	Dry/stuffy nose/congestion without discharge, better with sneezing, difficulty sneezing	Any Calcarea remedy has an affinity for bones, lymph nodes, circulation and polyps. Teeth are irregularly arranged and small in

		size, and the enamel is poor quality. #1 remedy for bone spurs. Multiple sprains, Discharges are usually green or yellow. This remedy is for chronic indications of ruta and rhus tox
Calc Phos		This remedy has an affinity for the bones, blood, lymph nodes and works on the nutrition of the body. Teeth are long, narrow and yellow, bones are long and straight, tired and nervous, rickets, weight loss, repetitive sore throat/bronchitis/colds
Calc Sulph	Nose discharge smelly/thick/blood-streaked/yellow, cold with headache, loss of smell, worse from drinking milk	This remedy has an affinity for the skin and glands. Eczema, pus formations, dizziness, sluggish, eye inflammation, ear discharges pus/blood/thick, croup, gout, worse walking/warm room/milk/movement /bath/night
Carb	Nose blocked, sneezing, difficulty	This remedy has an

o Veg	sneezing, hoarseness	affinity for the digestive system and the body's circulation. Lack of reaction, engorged veins, slow recovery of previous illness, sluggish, listless, indifferent
Dulc	Nose discharge thick and yellow, cold from wet weather	This remedy has an affinity for respiratory and digestive tract, lymphatic and muscular system, and the skin. Stuffy nose when exposed to cold, wet or rainy weather, catches a cold from air-conditioner, head cold in newborns
Euph	Eyes streaming/swollen/burning, nose discharge clear/non-irritating/watery, cough	This remedy has an affinity for the nose and the eyes. Pink eye, eyes clump together, worse heat/wind/night, better in the dark, measles
Hep Sul	Post-nasal drip, nose discharge smelly and yellow, sneezing especially when uncovered	This remedy is hypersensitive especially to touch and cold air, worse dry/cold weather/slightest draft, better with heat, craves sour things especially

			vinegar
Kali Bich	Nose discharge hard/crusty/post-nasal drip/dry/stuffy/congestion without discharge/smelly/stringy/sticky/thick/yellow/green, sinuses are blocked and painful, dry throat		This remedy has an affinity for mucus and the skin. Worse cold/2-3am/movement/drinking beer, better with heat, pains start and stop suddenly, aphthae in mouth, thirsty for beer, burning pain in stomach, sciatica left side, heel pain, ulcers, headaches from digestive issues
Kali Mur	Deafness from cold, nose discharge white		This remedy has an affinity for the ears and tonsils. Tubal discharge (ears)
Kali Sul	Nose discharge profuse and thick		This remedy has an affinity for the mucus and skin. Irritable, angry and obstinate, worse from heat/evening/resting, better from cold air/outdoors/walking, throbbing pains, bronchitis, asthma, eczema
Lyc	Nose discharge yellow, nose is dry, sinuses are blocked and painful, cold		This remedy has an affinity for liver and digestion, kidneys and

		with headache,	genitals, mucus and skin, and nervous system. Worse between 4-8pm, worse with heat, better with cool air, craving for sweets and oysters, ravenous appetite, flatulence, bloating after meals, doesn't like tight clothes on waist, abdomen is distended, red face after eating, migraine from poor digestion, bedwetting, nose stuffy with crusty mucus especially at night, sleep with mouth open, runny nose during day, anorexia in children, fear of new things, "devil at home and angel outside syndrome", lack of self-confidence
Mag Mur		Cold from swimming in the sea	This remedy has an affinity for the digestive and uterine system. Worse from salt (eating and being by sea) and drinking milk, better by pressure, tongue has teeth marks, constipation with hard stools like that of sheep

			droppings, migraines better with wrapping heat with warm compress
Merc Sol		Nose discharge bloody/burning/green/smelly/watery/yellow/green/sinuses are blocked and painful, sneezing, fever, cold with headache, hoarseness, loss of smell, worse with cold/heat/night	This remedy has an affinity for the digestive and renal systems with specific action on throat. Foul-smelling breath, gums are white/yellow color and ulcers in gums, tooth abscess, sores in mouth, intense thirst, thick tongue, salivate heavily, parotiditis, heavy perspiration especially at night and offensive in odor, ulcers, worse at night, known as "the human thermometer," shivering and goose-bumps
Nat Carb		Nose discharge smelly/thick/post-nasal drip	This remedy has an affinity for the nervous and digestive system. Worse from heat/cold/music/mental activity, better from motion, headaches from exposure to sun, diarrhea with urgency to go with yellow stools

		with orange pulp-like substances
Nat Mur	Eyes watery, nose discharge egg-white color/profuse/watery alternating with congestion/post-nasal drip, loss of smell and taste	This remedy can be summed up with three words: Malnutrition, dehydrated and weak. Worse being consoled, worse 10am, worse when at the ocean, loss of vital fluids will cause symptoms, discharge is clear and in large quantities, craves salt, eczema in the creases of joints/forehead/edge of scalp, herpetic rashes especially after illness, dry and cracked skin, chapped lips
Nitric Ac	Nose discharge bloody/burning/watery/dirty yellow/congested	This remedy has an affinity for the body's mucus. Worse from cold/noise/night, better from heat and riding in the car, prickling pains, craves fatty foods, lips are cracked in corners, anal fissures, plantar warts
Nux Vom	Eyes watery, nose discharge burning/watery/runny during day and stuffy at night, sinuses are blocked and painful, sneezing, cold with headache,	This remedy as an affinity for the nervous and digestive system. Irritable, cold,

	sore throat, worse after eating/getting up/morning, better with fresh air, cold from draught	hypersensitive, angry, worse after eating, better with sleep, tongue is yellow/white color, craves spicy and sour food, constipation, sneezing upon waking
Phos Ac		This remedy is severely exhausted especially because of emotional upset. Symptoms are caused by a loss of fluids, indifference to everything, fatigue, painless and orderless diarrhea, urine is milky colored, urine can also be clear in color, hair loss all over body
Phos	Nose discharge is blood-streaked/dry/stuffy/congested without discharge/profuse, loss of smell and taste, hoarseness	This remedy is highly sensitive especially to light, noises, and smells. Fear of thunderstorm, worse from cold/storms/left side, better from sleep, craves salt and cold drinks, midnight "snacker" especially around 3 am, #1 morning sickness remedy
Puls	Nose discharge is dry alternating with profuse/green/smelly/thick/watery/yell	This remedy has an affinity for the venous

		ow-green, sinuses are blocked and painful, sneezing especially in stuffy room, worse in stuffy room, better in fresh-open air	system and mucus. Changeable behavior, worse from heat, better from cold open air, thirstless, thick yellow/yellow-greenish discharge, worse after sunset, sleeps with feet uncovered
Sep		Nose discharge is/post-nasal drip/green/dirty yellow/yellow-green, loss of smell	This remedy has an affinity for the circulatory and nervous system. Hormonal imbalance. Sitting or kneeling for long periods causes fainting, worse before storm, better with exercise, feels like abdomen is heavy, flushes of heat in face, craves vinegar, and sour foods, worse 11 am
Sil		Nose discharge is dry/stuffy/congested/hard/crusty/smelly/thick, sinuses are blocked and painful, loss of smell and taste	This remedy has an affinity for the nervous system and is very malnourished. They are weak and demineralized. Worse cold and humid weather, better with heat, slinters (will push them out), fontanels stay open, perspire on

73

		head, abscess remedy, white spots on nails, weak nails/hair
Sul	Nose discharge is smelly and dirty yellow, nose is dry and itchy, sneezing, eye inflammation	This remedy has an affinity for the heart and skin. Worse standing still/heat of bed/water/11am, better perspiring/motion/dry weather, burning sensations all over body, eczema, craves sweets and open air, children look like they have a potbelly, children hate to take baths, wakes at 5am, vivid dreams, sleeps with feet uncovered

CONJUNCTIVITIS (PINK EYE)

REMEDIES:

Aconite, Allium Cepa, Apis, Argentrum Nitricum, Arsenicum Album, Belladonna, Bryonia, Calcarea Carb., Calcarea Sulph., Dulcamara, Euphrasia, Lycopodium, Mercurius Sol., Natrum Mur., Nitricum Acidum, Nux Vomica, Pulsatilla, Rhus Tox., Sepia, Silica, Sulphur, Zinc

Remedy	Symptom Differentiation	Keynote Differentiation
Acon	Eyes are aching/burning/red/sensitive to light, pink eye with cold,	This remedy has an affinity for the circulatory and nervous system. Worse extreme or

	pink eye from foreign body in eye or getting chilled	sudden cold/extreme heat/night, better with perspiration, rapid pulse, sudden high fever, red skin, intense thirst for large quantities of cold water, restlessness, anxiety, fear of death, croup cough
All Cep	Discharge is non-irritating/watery/profuse	This remedy has an affinity for the upper respiratory mucus, intestines and nervous system. Cough is loud/raspy/spasmodic, worse in evening/heat/heated room, better in cool or open air, whooping cough
Apis	Eyelids are swollen, eyes are burning/red/sore/stinging/stitching, worse heat	This remedy is known for swelling, burning pain, and jealousy. Worse from heat, better from cold, hot dry skin, inflammation
Arg Nit	Discharge is pus/smelly/yellow, eyelids are glued together and red, eyes are red and sensitive to light, better with cold and cold compresses	This remedy has an affinity for the nervous system and the mucus. Nervousness, "what-if," feels as if a thorn is stuck certain part of body, feels like head is expanding, feels squeezing sensation, worse from heat/eating candy/intellectual work/right side, better from fresh air and pressure, vertigo, anticipation anxiety (especially for tests),

			stomach ulcers
Ars		Eyes are burning/gritty (sand sensation)/sensitive to light	This remedy has an affinity for mucus, kidneys liver, adrenal glands and the nervous system. This remedy can be summed up in three words: weak, restless and cold (temperature-wise). Burning pains, worse 1-3am and from the cold, thirsty for small amounts of cold water, fear of death, food-poisoning
Bell		Eyes are bloodshot/burning/dry/sensitive to light/watering, pink eye with cold, worse heat and light	Symptoms usually have sudden and violent onset, local congestion of blood (example face is red), the congested area is usually hot, children usually convulse when they have a fever
Bry		Eyes are dry and sore, soreness is worse moving the eyes	Very thirsty especially if during a fever, sinuses are very dry (hint to remember: if dry think "bry"), pressure headaches that usually travel from forehead to occiput, or can start from left eye and move to the back of the head
Calc Carb		Discharge is pus, eyelids are glued together and gritty, eyes are gritty/sensitive to light/watering, pink eye with cold	Any Calcarea remedy has an affinity for bones, lymph nodes, circulation and polyps. They sweat profusely on head, babies teethe late, walk slow and are lazy, large appetite,

		remember the four F's: fat, fair skin, fainting, and fearful. If Ruta and Rhus Tox have stopped working, this remedy can be thought of. For chronic indications of pulsatilla
Calc Sulph	Discharge is pus/thick/yellow	This remedy has an affinity for the skin and glands. Eczema, pus formations, dizziness, sluggish, eye inflammation, ear discharges pus/blood/thick, croup, gout, worse walking/warm room/milk/movement/bath/night
Dulc	Pink eye with cold and from cold/wet weather	This remedy has an affinity for respiratory and digestive tract, lymphatic and muscular system, and the skin. Stuffy nose when exposed to cold, wet or rainy weather, catches a cold from air-conditioner, head cold in newborns
Euph	Discharge is watery and burning, eyelids are burning/red/swollen/sensitive to light/watering, pink eye with cold, worse light and wind	This remedy has an affinity for the nose and the eyes. Pink eye, eyes clump together, worse heat/wind/night, better in the dark, measles
Lyc	Discharge is pus, eyelids glued together, sensitive to light, eyes stitching	This remedy has an affinity for liver and digestion, kidneys and genitals, mucus and skin, and nervous system. Worse

		between 4-8pm, worse with heat, better with cool air, craving for sweets and oysters, ravenous appetite, flatulence, bloating after meals, doesn't like tight clothes on waist, abdomen is distended, red face after eating, migraine from poor digestion, bedwetting, nose stuffy with crusty mucus especially at night, sleep with mouth open, runny nose during day, anorexia in children, fear of new things, "devil at home and angel outside syndrome", lack of self-confidence
Merc Sol	Discharge is pus, sensitive to light, eyes are watering, pink eye with cold, worse heat, even heat of the bed is worse	This remedy has an affinity for the digestive and renal systems with specific action on throat. Foul-smelling breath, gums are white/yellow color and ulcers in gums, tooth abscess, sores in mouth, intense thirst, thick tongue, salivate heavily, parotiditis, heavy perspiration especially at night and offensive in odor, ulcers, worse at night, known as "the human thermometer," shivering and goose-bumps
Nat Mur	Eyes are gritty/sensitive to light/watering	This remedy can be summed up with three words: Malnutrition, dehydrated and

		weak. Worse being consoled, worse 10am, worse when at the ocean, loss of vital fluids will cause symptoms, discharge is clear and in large quantities, craves salt, eczema in the creases of joints/forehead/edge of scalp, herpetic rashes especially after illness, dry and cracked skin, chapped lips,
Nit Ac	Eyelids are swollen, eyes are watering	This remedy has an affinity for the body's mucus. Worse from cold/noise/night, better from heat and riding in the car, prickling pains, craves fatty foods, lips are cracked in corners, anal fissures, plantar warts
Nux Vom	Sensitive to light	This remedy as an affinity for the nervous and digestive system. Irritable, cold, hypersensitive, angry, worse after eating, better with sleep, tongue is yellow/white color, craves spicy and sour food, constipation, sneezing upon waking
Puls	Discharge is pus/smelly/thick/yellow, eyelids are itching, eyes are aching/burning/itching/watering, pink eye with cold, better cold/bath/fresh air, worse	This remedy has an affinity for the venous system and mucus. Changeable behavior, worse from heat, better from cold open air, thirstless, thick yellow/yellow-greenish

		warm room and evening	discharge, worse after sunset
Rhus Tox		Eyelids are glued together/itching/swollen, eyes are sensitive to light/sire/watering, worse moving eyes, pink eye from cold/wet weather	This remedy has an affinity for the skin, mucus and the nervous system. Better with slow motion and changing of position, shivers when slights part of body is uncovered, perspiration all over body except the face, sprains and dislocations, worse 4-5am and 7pm, intense thirst for cold water or milk
Sep		Eyelids are glued together and swollen, eyes are burning, worse evening/reading/after walk	This remedy has an affinity for the circulatory and nervous system. Hormonal imbalance. Sitting or kneeling for long periods causes fainting, worse before storm, better with exercise, feels like abdomen is heavy, flushes of heat in face, craves vinegar, and sour foods, worse 11 am
Sil		Discharge is yellow, worse cold air, pink eye from foreign body in eye	This remedy has an affinity for the nervous system and is very malnourished. They are weak and demineralized. Worse cold and humid weather, better with heat, slinters (will push them out), fontanels stay open, perspire on head, abscess remedy, white spots on nails, weak nails/hair

Sul	Eyelids are burning/itching/red, eyes burning/gritty/stitching, worse washing eyes	This remedy has an affinity for the heart and skin. Worse standing still/heat of bed/water/11am, better perspiring/motion/dry weather, burning sensations all over body, eczema, craves sweets and open air, children look like they have a potbelly, children hate to take baths
Zinc	Eyes burning/gritty/sore, worse at night	Restless leg syndrome, worse alcohol especially wine, better with any discharge

CONSTIPATION

REMEDIES:

Aesculus, Alumina, Calcarea Carb., Cuasticum, Hepar Sulph, Kali Carb., Lycopodium, Magnesia Mur., Natrum Mur., Nux Vomica, Opium, Pulsatilla, Sepia, Silica, Sulphur, Zinc

Remedy	Symptom Differentiation	Keynote Differentiation
Aesc	Stools are hard/large/burning after passing, straining	Major hip remedy, generally better by creating better circulation such as exercise, cold, hemorrhoid remedy
Alu	No desire to pass stool, stool soft, constipation from being bottle-fed	This remedy has an affinity for the skin and mucus. Weakness,

		and weaning	dryness, wrinkled, afraid of sharp instruments and blood, extreme constipation, worse in morning and after eating potatoes, better open air and wearing warm clothes
Calc Carb		Stools are hard at first/large/pale/sour-smelling, better being constipated	Any Calcarea remedy has an affinity for bones, lymph nodes, circulation and polyps. They sweat profusely on head, babies teethe late, walk slow and are lazy, large appetite, remember the four F's: fat, fair skin, fainting, and fearful. If Ruta and Rhus Tox have stopped working, this remedy can be thought of. For chronic indications of pulsatilla
Caust		Desire to pass stool is ineffectual, stitching pain, better passing stool while standing	This remedy can be summed up in two words: weakness and paralysis. Worse cold/3-4am/when thinking about symptoms, better with heat and humidity and cold water, warts under the nails, crave smoked

		foods
Hep Sul	Stool is soft	This remedy is hypersensitive especially to touch and cold air, worse dry/cold weather/slightest draft, better with heat, craves sour things especially vinegar
Kali Carb	Stool is hard and large, unfinished feeling after passing stool	This remedy has an affinity for the nervous, digestive and respiratory system with specific action on lungs, mucus and blood. Weary, anemic and tired complexion, swelling inside upper eyelid, perspire easily, hypersensitive to noise and touch, anxiety, absent-minded, worse 2-5am, asthma which is better by sitting forward with elbows on knees, #1 stomach ulcer remedy, PMS remedy, flatulence
Lyc	Desire to pass stool is ineffectual, hard and knotty stool, flatulence	This remedy has an affinity for liver and digestion, kidneys and genitals, mucus and skin, and nervous

			system. Worse between 4-8pm, worse with heat, better with cool air, craving for sweets and oysters, ravenous appetite, flatulence, bloating after meals, doesn't like tight clothes on waist, abdomen is distended, red face after eating, migraine from poor digestion, bedwetting, nose stuffy with crusty mucus especially at night, sleep with mouth open, runny nose during day, anorexia in children
Mag Mur		Desire to pass stool is ineffectual, stools are hard/crumbling/knotty/large/passed with difficulty/look like sheep dropping/small balls, strain to pass stool, worse drinking milk especially cow's milk	This remedy has an affinity for the digestive and uterine system. Worse from salt (eating and being by sea) and drinking milk, better by pressure, tongue has teeth marks, constipation with hard stools like that of sheep droppings, migraines better with wrapping heat with warm compress

Nat Mur	Desire to pass stool is ineffectual, stools are like sheep droppings/small balls/crumbling, straining, unfinished feeling after passing stool	This remedy can be summed up with three words: Malnutrition, dehydrated and weak. Worse being consoled, worse 10am, worse when at the ocean, loss of vital fluids will cause symptoms, discharge is clear and in large quantities, craves salt, eczema in the creases of joints/forehead/edge of scalp, herpetic rashes especially after illness, dry and cracked skin, chapped lips,
Nux Vom	Constant desire to pass stool, desire is ineffectual, stool is hard and large, unfinished feeling after passing stool, constipation from over-heating and weaning, constipation alternating with diarrhea	This remedy as an affinity for the nervous and digestive system. Irritable, cold, hypersensitive, angry, worse after eating, better with sleep, tongue is yellow/white color, craves spicy and sour food, constipation, sneezing upon waking
Op	No desire to pass stool, stools are black balls/hard/like sheep droppings/recede/small balls, unfinished feeling after passing stool,	This remedy has an affinity for the brain. Coma-like sleep, dark red or purple face, hot

	constipation from bottle-feeding and weaning	perspiration, slow breathing, slow pulse, hypersensitivity of ears, worse from heat/fear/strong emotion, better from cold, absence of pain
Puls	Changeable stools	This remedy has an affinity for the venous system and mucus. Changeable behavior, worse from heat, better from cold open air, thirstless, thick yellow/yellow-greenish discharge, worse after sunset
Sep	Abdomen and stomach feels full, desire to pass stool is ineffectual, stools are hard and large, straining	This remedy has an affinity for the circulatory and nervous system. Hormonal imbalance. Sitting or kneeling for long periods causes fainting, worse before storm, better with exercise, feels like abdomen is heavy, flushes of heat in face, craves vinegar, and sour foods, worse 11 am,
Sil	Desire to pass stool is ineffectual, stool is burning/hard/knotty/large/recede,	This remedy has an affinity for the nervous system and is very

		straining	malnourished. They are weak and demineralized. Worse cold and humid weather, better with heat, slinters (will push them out), fontanels stay open, perspire on head, abscess remedy, white spots on nails, weak nails/hair
Sul			This remedy has an affinity for the heart and skin. Worse standing still/heat of bed/water/11am, better perspiring/motion/dry weather, burning sensations all over body, eczema, craves sweets and open air, children look like they have a potbelly, children hate to take baths
Zinc		Constipation in newborns	Restless leg syndrome, worse alcohol especially wine, better with any discharge

CONVULSIONS

REMEDIES:

Belladonna, Cina, Cuprum, Stramonium

Remedy	Symptom Differentiation	Keynote Differentiation
Bell	Convulsions during teething	Symptoms usually have sudden and violent onset, local congestion of blood (example face is red), the congested area is usually hot, children usually convulse when they have a fever
Cin	Convulsions during teething/ worms	Convulsions beginning on one side of the face, attack stops and begins at the same time, breathing slows down, urine incontinence, do not like to be touched or looked at, large circles under the eyes, sickly appearance, yawn frequently, grinding of teeth, restless sleep, frequent rubbing of nose and scratching of nostrils, constant hunger that is not easily satiable, pain in belly-button better by lying on abdomen, worse

			during new moon and full moon, better lying on stomach/abdomen, presence of round worms, teething
	Cup	Convulsions during teething/worms/suppressed anger, blue lips, cold hands and feet	This remedy has an affinity for the muscular system. Spasmodic pain begins and ends suddenly, convulsions, blue face, violent cramping, whooping cough, better drinking a sip of cold water, violent diarrhea with cramping pains
	Stram	Convulsions from over-excitement/fever/rage	This remedy has an affinity for the brain and the nervous system. Worse in dark/shinny and bright objects/being alone, better from soft light and being around people, severe and violent convulsions, incoherent talkativeness, hallucinations, nightmares, swollen tongue, doesn't like the sight of liquids, spasmodic and suffocative cough,

		bright red rash

COUGH

REMEDIES:

Aconite, Allium Cepa, Antimonium Tart., Arnica, Arsenicum Album, Baryt Carb., Belladonna, Bryonia, Calcarea Carb., Calcarea Phos., Calcarea Sulph., Carbo Veg., Causticum, Chamomilla, Cina, Coccus Cacti, Conium, Cuprum, Drosera, Dulcamara, Euphrasia, Ferrum Metallicum, Hepar Sulphur, Ignatia, Ipecacuanha, Kali Bich., Kali Carb., Kali Mur., Kali Sulph., Lachesis, Lycopodium, Mercurius Sol., Natrum Mur., Natrum Sulph., Nux Vomica, Opium, Phosphoricum Acidum, Phosphorus, Pulsatilla, Rhus Tox., Rumex, Sepia, Silica, Spongia, Staphysagria, Sulphur, Veratrum Album

Remedy	Symptom Differentiation	Keynote Differentiation
Acon	Fast breathing, cough is barking/dry/irritating/short, fever, hoarseness, worse dry and cold weather/night/during fever, cough from cold and dry wind	This remedy has an affinity for the circulatory and nervous system. Worse extreme or sudden cold/extreme heat/night, better with perspiration, rapid pulse, sudden high fever, red skin, intense thirst for large quantities of cold water, restlessness, anxiety, fear of death, croup cough
All Cep	Cough is hacking/worse cold air/irritating/painful, tickling in larynx, hoarseness, hacking, better warm room	This remedy has an affinity for the upper respiratory mucus, intestines and nervous system. Cough is

			loud/raspy/spasmodic, worse in evening/heat/heated room, better in cool or open air, whooping cough
Ant Tart		Breathing is asthmatic/difficult/fast/rattling/loud, vomiting with or after cough, whooping cough, difficult to bring up mucus, sleepy with cough	This remedy has an affinity for the respiratory system and the skin. This remedy can be summed up with three words: exhaustion, paleness, and sleepiness. Spitting behavior, grasps for other people
Arn		Pain in chest from cough, bloodshot eyes from cough, nosebleed from cough, worse crying	This remedy has an affinity for the muscles, capillaries and cellular tissues. Contusions, stiffness, muscular pain, feel that bed is too hard, worse from slightest touch/jolt/movement/damp cold, better from lying with head lower than feet, #1 trauma remedy/accidents/falls/hemorrhaging, given to stop bleeding. If you have children, you will give this remedy to your child several times throughout their childhood. For falls and

		bleeding, give the highest potency you have.
Ars	Breathing is fast and wheezing, cough is dry (especially at night)/exhausting/hacking (especially from tickling in larynx)/loose/tormenting/produces large amount of mucus. Mucus is frothy and tastes salty, sweating from coughing, better from hot drinks and sitting up, worse cold/evening/fever/lying down/night (especially after midnight)	This remedy has an affinity for mucus, kidneys liver, adrenal glands and the nervous system. This remedy can be summed up in three words: weak, restless and cold (temperature-wise). Burning pains, worse 1-3am and from the cold, thirsty for small amounts of cold water, fear of death, food-poisoning
Bar C	Cough worse at night	This remedy has an affinity for the mental development, arteries, and lymphatic system. Late development/milestones, shy, worse cold/humid/thinking about problems
Bell	Fast or slow breathing, cough is barking/dry/exhausting/hard/hollow/irritating/racking/tormenting/violent, sharp pain in chest from coughing, worse deep breathing and night, cough from getting chilled	Symptoms usually have sudden and violent onset, local congestion of blood (example face is red), the congested area is usually hot, children usually convulse when they have a fever

Bry	Breathing is fast, cough is dry/disturbs sleep/irritating/painful/racking/vomiting with or after cough, pain in chest and stomach from cough, cough with splitting headache, better from fresh air, worse from deep breathing and on the right lung	Very thirsty especially if during a fever, sinuses are very dry (hint to remember: if dry think "bry"), pressure headaches that usually travel from forehead to occiput, or can start from left eye and move to the back of the head
Calc Carb	Cough is dry in evening and loose in morning, cough produces a large amount of mucus, and is lumpy/smelly/tastes sweet and sour/tough/yellow, worse during fever and playing piano	Any Calcarea remedy has an affinity for bones, lymph nodes, circulation and polyps. They sweat profusely on head, babies teethe late, walk slow and are lazy, large appetite, remember the four F's: fat, fair skin, fainting, and fearful. If Ruta and Rhus Tox have stopped working, this remedy can be thought of
Calc Phos	Mucus is yellow, cough during teething	This remedy has an affinity for the bones, blood, lymph nodes and works on the nutrition of the body. Teeth are long, narrow and yellow, bones are long and straight, tired and nervous, rickets, weight loss, repetitive sore throat/bronchitis/colds

Calc Sulph	Cough is dry, large amount of mucus which is lumpy and yellow	This remedy has an affinity for the skin and glands. Eczema, pus formations, dizziness, sluggish, eye inflammation, ear discharges pus/blood/thick, croup, gout, worse walking/warm room/milk/movement/bath/night
Carbo Veg	Fast breathing and wheezing, cough is in fits/racking/suffocative/violent/whooping, mucus is green, dry heaving (retching), hoarseness, worse evening before midnight	This remedy has an affinity for the digestive system and the body's circulation. Lack of reaction, engorged veins, slow recovery of previous illness, sluggish, listless, indifferent
Caust	Cough is constant/distressing/exhausting/hollow/racking/rattling/violent/tormenting/wakens from sleep, mucus is difficult to bring up and swallows it, raw pain in chest from cough, hoarseness, better from sipping cold water, worse from bending head forward/breathing cold air/warmth of bed/lying down	This remedy can be summed up in two words: weakness and paralysis. Worse cold/3-4am/when thinking about symptoms, better with heat and humidity and cold water, warts under the nails, crave smoked foods
Cham	Cough is dry at night and irritating, mucus tastes bitter, worse at night	This remedy has an affinity for the digestive system. Hypersensitive to pain, pain feels

			intolerable, numbness, irritable, angry, moody, hateful, exhausted from teething, insomnia, one cheek is red and hot while other is pale and cold, worse from anger/9pm and 12am/heat(toothache), better from being carried or riding in car
	Cina	Dry heaving (retching) from cough	Convulsions beginning on one side of the face, attack stops and begins at the same time, breathing slows down, urine incontinence, do not like to be touched or looked at, large circles under the eyes, sickly appearance, yawn frequently, grinding of teeth, restless sleep, frequent rubbing of nose and scratching of nostrils, constant hunger that is not easily satiable, pain in belly-button better by lying on abdomen, worse during new moon and full moon, better lying on stomach/abdomen, presence of round worms, teething
	Cocc C	Coughing fits from ticking in larynx,	This remedy has an

	mucus is stringy/large amount/thick, worse 11:30pm/morning/heat, better in cold room and drinking sip of cold water, better fresh air, whooping cough, spasmodic cough, chocking cough, dry throat,	affinity for the respiratory mucus and kidneys.
Con	Cough is dry/irritating/violent, mucus is difficult to bring up and swallows it, better from sitting up, worse deep breathing/evening/lying down	This remedy has an affinity for the nervous system and lymph nodes. Dizziness from turning head, tearing from light (photophobia), cannot tolerate light, profuse sweating while sleeping, hard nodes in breasts, mastitis, worse from cold and alcohol, better from dangling legs, pains are knife-like, stools and gas feel cold, intense craving for salt, very thirsty
Cup	Breathing difficult and fast, cough is in long/uninterrupted/irregular fits/violent/whooping, worse from cold air, better from sips of cold water	This remedy has an affinity for the muscular system. Spasmodic pain begins and ends suddenly, convulsions, blue face, violent cramping, whooping cough, better drinking a sip of cold water, violent diarrhea with cramping pains
Dros	Cough is dry/quick/tearing/spasmodic/hacki	This remedy has an affinity for the mucus of

	ng/irritating/barking, tickling in larynx, wheezes when inhaling, whooping cough, breathing is difficult in between coughing fits, face turns blue from coughing, vomiting from cough, mucus is bloody, nosebleeds from cough, abdominal pain from cough which is better with pressure, worse from drinking/lying down/talking/after midnight, fast and difficult breathing, pain in chest from cough, dry heaving (retching), cough from measles	the larynx and bronchi, as well as the lymphatic system and bones. Worse at night/heat of bed/laughing/singing, better from moving
Dulc	Rattling, worse wet and damp weather	This remedy has an affinity for respiratory and digestive tract, lymphatic and muscular system, and the skin. Stuffy nose when exposed to cold, wet or rainy weather, catches a cold from air-conditioner, head cold in newborns
Euph	Cough in daytime only, worse in morning, better from lying down, large amount of mucus	This remedy has an affinity for the nose and the eyes. Pink eye, eyes clump together, worse heat/wind/night, better in the dark, measles
Fer M	Cough in fits, better from walking slowly, worse from movement	This remedy has an affinity for the blood and spleen. Mothers are never the same after

			childbirth. Pale and blush very easily. Weak, tired, sensitive to cold, cannot make effort, urinate involuntarily when coughing or sneezing or when children play, throbbing headache with hammering pain
Hep Sul		Cough is barking/dry (especially at night)/hacking/after dinner/irritating/suffocative/violent/vomiting after, mucus is sticky/thick/large amount/yellow, dry heaving (retching), sweating and vomiting from cough, hoarseness, worse from cold/evening in bed/before midnight/uncovering, cough from cold and dry wind	This remedy is hypersensitive especially to touch and cold air, worse dry/cold weather/slightest draft, better with heat, craves sour things especially vinegar
Ign		Cough is dry/hacking (especially in evening when lying down)/irritating/violent, pain in chest when coughing is racking/short/stitching, worse evening in bed	This remedy is hypersensitive on all organs and senses especially sight and hearing. Very sensitive emotionally especially to sad events, spasms, uncoordinated, sensitive to any sort of excitement or pain, nervous behavior, sighing, fainting, moody, outbreaks of anger, cries easily, irritability, weakness, feels like lump

		in throat, migraines feel like nails in head, worse 11am/sad news/being consoled/strong smells, better from heat and good time with company, nervous breakdown
Ipecac	Breathing is fast/difficult/wheezing, cough is chocking/dry/in fits/irritating/whooping, vomiting after cough, mucus is bloody, blue face/dry heaving (retching)/nausea/vomiting from coughing	This remedy has an affinity for the digestive and respiratory system. Hemorrhaging bright red blood, profuse saliva, not thirsty at all, disgusted by food, persistent and violent nausea, vomit is sticky and does not relieve nausea, stools are fermented like yeast, cough with suffocation, large amount of mucus
Kali Bich	Mucus is difficult to bring up/sticky/ropy/stringy/thick/tough, sore and bruised pain in chest from cough, hoarseness, worse eating and upon waking in morning	This remedy has an affinity for mucus and the skin. Worse cold/2-3am/movement/drinking beer, better with heat, pains start and stop suddenly, aphthae in mouth, thirsty for beer, burning pain in stomach, sciatica left side, heel pain, ulcers, headaches from digestive issues
Kali	Wheezing, cough disturbs sleep/dry/hard/irritating/racking/v	This remedy has an affinity for the nervous,

Carb	iolent/wakens up from sleep, cutting pain in chest from cough, nausea, worse from cold/deep breathing/evening/fever/heat/lying down/night, cough from getting chilled	digestive and respiratory system with specific action on lungs, mucus and blood. Weary, anemic and tired complexion, swelling inside upper eyelid, perspire easily, hypersensitive to noise and touch, anxiety, absent-minded, worse 2-5am, asthma which is better by sitting forward with elbows on knees, #1 stomach ulcer remedy, PMS remedy, flatulence
Kali Mur	Cough is short and hard	This remedy has an affinity for the ears and tonsils. Tubal discharge (ears)
Kali Sul	Whooping and rattling cough, mucus is difficult to bring up/swallows it/yellow, worse at night/warm room/stuffy room/heat	This remedy has an affinity for the mucus and skin. Irritable, angry and obstinate, worse from heat/evening/resting, better from cold air/outdoors/walking, throbbing pains, bronchitis, asthma, eczema
Lach	Cough as soon as deep sleep/dry/hacking/ticking in larynx/irritating/violent, worse	This remedy has an affinity for the nervous system and blood. Bruising, hemorrhaging,

		evening in bed/night/touch	blotchy face, talkative, suspicious, jealous, spiteful, depression, worse from discharges that are delayed or insufficient/being touched/sun/heat/sleeping/tight clothes/left side, better from discharge that finally comes out, insomnia (especially before midnight), dreams of ghosts, dead people, coffins, difficulty swallowing, sinusitis, apnea, hot flushes in head, ulcers, bed sores
	Lyc	Breathing is fast and difficult, cough is constant/disturbs sleep/dry/irritating, mucus is green/large amount/tastes salty/white/yellow, better from hot drinks, worse during evening in bed/lying down/night/going to sleep	This remedy has an affinity for liver and digestion, kidneys and genitals, mucus and skin, and nervous system. Worse between 4-8pm, worse with heat, better with cool air, craving for sweets and oysters, ravenous appetite, flatulence, bloating after meals, doesn't like tight clothes on waist, abdomen is distended, red face after eating, migraine from poor digestion, bedwetting, nose stuffy with crusty

			mucus especially at night, sleep with mouth open, runny nose during day, anorexia in children, fear of new things, "devil at home and angel outside syndrome", lack of self-confidence
Nat Mur		Cough is dry/hacking/tickling in larynx/irritating, mucus is egg-white like/transparent/white, worse during fever	This remedy can be summed up with three words: Malnutrition, dehydrated and weak. Worse being consoled, worse 10am, worse when at the ocean, loss of vital fluids will cause symptoms, discharge is clear and in large quantities, craves salt, eczema in the creases of joints/forehead/edge of scalp, herpetic rashes especially after illness, dry and cracked skin, chapped lips
Nat Sulph		Cough during daytime only, mucus is green, worse from wet and damp weather	This remedy has an affinity for digestive, respiratory and nervous system, with effects on the joints and skin, worse from cold and humidity, intense thirst especially for cold drinks, watery stool that squirt out

		especially in the morning, bronchitis, asthma in children, holds chest when coughing
Nux Vom	Difficult breathing, cough is dry and irritating, hacking produces vomit, better from hot drinks, worse from cold/cold air/eating/fever/morning/upon waking in morning	This remedy as an affinity for the nervous and digestive system. Irritable, cold, hypersensitive, angry, worse after eating, better with sleep, tongue is yellow/white color, craves spicy and sour food, constipation, sneezing upon waking
Op	Breathing is difficult and slow, snoring, worse during sleep/falling asleep/warmth of bed/upon waking in morning	This remedy has an affinity for the brain. Coma-like sleep, dark red or purple face, hot perspiration, slow breathing, slow pulse, hypersensitivity of ears, worse from heat/fear/strong emotion, better from cold, absence of pain
Phos Ac	Cough is dry/irritating/violent	This remedy is severely exhausted especially because of emotional upset. Symptoms are caused by a loss of fluids, indifference to everything, fatigue, painless and orderless

			diarrhea, urine is milky colored, urine can also be clear in color, hair loss all over body
Phos		Difficult breathing, cough is dry at night/tickling in larynx/irritating/racking/tight/violent, mucus is green/large amount/tastes sweet and salty/white/yellow, burning pain in chest from cough, sweating from cough, better sitting up, worse change of temperature/fever/reading aloud	This remedy is highly sensitive especially to light, noises, and smells. Fear of thunderstorm, worse from cold/storms/left side, better from sleep, craves salt and cold drinks, midnight "snacker" especially around 3 am, #1 morning sickness remedy
Puls		Cough is constant/dry (especially in evening and during fever)/loose in morning/in fits/irritating/racking/violent, mucus is sticky/green/in large amount/difficult to bring up/tastes bitter and salty/yellow/yellow-green, nausea with cough, better with fresh air and sitting up, worse from getting hot/evening/morning/night/physical exertion/stuffy room, cough from measles	This remedy has an affinity for the venous system and mucus. Changeable behavior, worse from heat, better from cold open air, thirstless, thick yellow/yellow-greenish discharge, worse after sunset, sleeps with feet uncovered
Rhus Tox		Cough is irritating and short, worse becoming cold and uncovering hands, cough from swimming in cold water	This remedy has an affinity for the skin, mucus and the nervous system. Better with slow motion and changing of

		position, shivers when slights part of body is uncovered, perspiration all over body except the face, sprains and dislocations, worse 4-5am and 7pm, intense thirst for cold water or milk
Rum	Cough is dry/continuous/itching and tickling in sternum area/in fits/irritating, sore/bruised/stitching pain in chest from cough, worse breathing cold air/cold/fresh air/left side/talking/uncovering/walking	This remedy has an affinity for the respiratory and intestinal mucus, and skin. Sensitive to cold, worse breathing cold air/undressing/evening, better from heat,
Sep	Fast breathing, cough is constant (especially when lying down)/disturbs sleep/dry/exhausting/hacking (especially when lying down)/irritating/ratting/loose/violent, mucus is white/yellow/tastes salty/large amount, better sitting up, worse during evening in bed/lying down/night	This remedy has an affinity for the circulatory and nervous system. Hormonal imbalance. Sitting or kneeling for long periods causes fainting, worse before storm, better with exercise, feels like abdomen is heavy, flushes of heat in face, craves vinegar, and sour foods, worse 11 am
Sil	Cough is irritating, mucus is lumpy and yellow, worse becoming cold/uncovering feet/upon waking in morning	This remedy has an affinity for the nervous system and is very malnourished. They are weak and demineralized. Worse cold and humid

		weather, better with heat, slinters (will push them out), fontanels stay open, perspire on head, abscess remedy, white spots on nails, weak nails/hair
Spon	Cough is dry/croup/wheezing/sounds like a saw cutting piece of wood/barking/hollow/irritating, burning mucus, burning pain in chest from cough, better drinking or eating	This remedy has an affinity of the respiratory mucus, glands, and lymphatic system. Worse at night/head lowered/inside hot room, better from hot drinks and raising head, dryness of nose and larynx
Staph	Cough is irritating, cough from suppressed anger	This remedy has an affinity for the urinary and genital system as well as the skin. Hypersensitive to emotions, excitable, irritated easily, obsessed about sexual ideas, burning/frequent/dripping urination, eczema with severe itching, styes especially on upper eyelids
Sul	Fast breathing, cough is dry (especially at night)/loose by day/disturbs sleep/irritating/painful/racking/suffocative, chest is congested, larynx feels raw, mucus is green, worse	This remedy has an affinity for the heart and skin. Worse standing still/heat of bed/water/11am, better perspiring/motion/dry

	evening/lying down/night	weather, burning sensations all over body, eczema, craves sweets and open air, children look like they have a potbelly, children hate to take baths
Verat A	Breathing is difficult, cough is deep	This remedy has an affinity for the digestive and nervous system. Weakness, collapsing, exhaustion, cold sweats on forehead, coldness all over body, burning inside of body, large amounts of vomiting/diarrhea/perspiration, worse cold and humid weather, better heat, cholera-like diarrhea

CRADLE CAP

REMEDIES:

Calcarea Carb., Lycopodium, Sulphur, Thuja, Coconut Oil (Non-homeopathic)

Remedy	Symptom Differentiation	Keynote Differentiation
Calc Carb	Cradle cap from profuse sweating on head and scalp	Any Calcarea remedy has an affinity for bones, lymph nodes, circulation and polyps. They sweat

		profusely on head, babies teethe late, walk slow and are lazy, large appetite, remember the four F's: fat, fair skin, fainting, and fearful. If Ruta and Rhus Tox have stopped working, this remedy can be thought of. For chronic indications of pulsatilla
Lyc		This remedy has an affinity for liver and digestion, kidneys and genitals, mucus and skin, and nervous system. Worse between 4-8pm, worse with heat, better with cool air, craving for sweets and oysters, ravenous appetite, flatulence, bloating after meals, doesn't like tight clothes on waist, abdomen is distended, red face after eating, migraine from poor digestion, bedwetting, nose stuffy with crusty mucus especially at night, sleep with mouth open, runny nose during day, anorexia in children
Sul		This remedy has an affinity for the heart and skin. Worse standing still/heat of bed/water/11am, better

			perspiring/motion/dry weather, burning sensations all over body, eczema, craves sweets and open air, children look like they have a potbelly, children hate to take baths
Thuja			This remedy has an affinity for the heart and skin. Worse standing still/heat of bed/water/11am, better perspiring/motion/dry weather, burning sensations all over body, eczema, craves sweets and open air, children look like they have a potbelly, children hate to take baths
Coconut Oil		For best results keep refrigerated and when ready to use, rub small amount in palm of hands to liquefy	Coconut Oil has anti-fungal properties. If applied directly onto scalp, within a few minutes, scales can be combed out.

CUTS
REMEDIES:
Calendula, Hypericum, Staphysagria

Remedy	Symptom Differentiation	Keynote Differentiation
Calen	To heal clean cuts not infected yet	Healing of wounds
Hyp	Infected and deep cuts, pain is shooting and cutting	This remedy has an affinity for the nervous system, painful scars, worse after having tooth pulled

Staph	Deep clean cuts, stab wound	This remedy has an affinity for the urinary and genital system as well as the skin. Hypersensitive to emotions, excitable, irritated easily, obsessed about sexual ideas, burning/frequent/dripping urination, eczema with severe itching, styes especially on upper eyelids

DIAPER RASH

REMEDIES:

Apis, Petroleum, Rhus Tox., Sulphur

Remedy	Symptom Differentiation	Keynote Differentiation
Apis	Red, hot, shiny, sore, better from uncovering, worse from bathing/washing/heat/touch	This remedy is known for swelling, burning pain, and jealousy. Worse from heat, better from cold, hot dry skin, inflammation
Petro	Bleeding, cracked, dry, itchy, red, weepy, worse in folds of skin	This remedy has an affinity for the skin and digestive mucus. Seasickness, worse from cold/winter/motion sickness, better in summer and heat, motion sickness better closing eyes, hands chapped (especially in winter), intense hunger and thirst,

		diarrhea only in morning
Rhus Tox	Burning, flaky, itching, better from uncovering, worse from cold	This remedy has an affinity for the skin, mucus and the nervous system. Better with slow motion and changing of position, shivers when slights part of body is uncovered, perspiration all over body except the face, sprains and dislocations, worse 4-5am and 7pm, intense thirst for cold water or milk
Sul	Burning, bleeding, hot, itching, red, raw, better from uncovering, worse from bathing/washing/heat	This remedy has an affinity for the heart and skin. Worse standing still/heat of bed/water/11am, better perspiring/motion/dry weather, burning sensations all over body, eczema, craves sweets and open air, children look like they have a potbelly, children hate to take baths

DIARRHEA

REMEDIES:

Antimonium Crudum, Apis, Argentrum Nitricum, Arsenicum Album, Borax, Bryonia, Calcarea Carb., Calcarea Phos., Chamomilla, China, Colchicum, Colocynthis, Dulcamara, Ferrum Metallicum, Gelsemium, Hepar Sulph., Ipecacuanha, Magnesia Carb., Magnesia Mur., Mercurius Corrivus, Mercurius Sol., Natrum Mur., Natrum Sulph., Nux Vomica, Petroleum, Phosphoricum Acidum, Phosphorus, Podophylum, Pulsatilla, Rheum, Rhus Tox., Silica, Sulphur, Sulphuricum Acidum, Veratrum Album

Remedy	Symptom Differentiation	Keynote Differentiation
Ant Crud	Diarrhea is watery, worse after sour wine/being over-heated/over-eating	This remedy has an affinity for the digestive tract, especially the stomach, and the skin. Tongue has thick white coating, thrush, burping, watery diarrhea, impetigo, warts, thick and hard nails, worse cold bath/radiating heat/over-eating
Apis	Painless diarrhea	This remedy is known for swelling, burning pain, and jealousy. Worse from heat, better from cold, hot dry skin, inflammation
Arg Nit	Diarrhea is green/smelly/watery/gassy/vomiting with diarrhea, worse after drinking (almost immediately)/night/sugar or sweets, diarrhea from anticipation anxiety (especially test)/excitement/weaning	This remedy has an affinity for the nervous system and the mucus. Nervousness, "what-if," feels as if a thorn is stuck certain part of body, feels like head is expanding, feels squeezing sensation, worse from heat/eating candy/intellectual work/right side, better from fresh air and pressure, vertigo, anticipation anxiety (especially for tests), stomach

			ulcers
Ars		Diarrhea is painful/burning/smelly/watery/exhausting/hands and feet cold/nausea/sweating, worse from cold/after drinking/eating/cold food/fruit/after midnight/night/ice cream/food poisoning	This remedy has an affinity for mucus, kidneys liver, adrenal glands and the nervous system. This remedy can be summed up in three words: weak, restless and cold (temperature-wise). Burning pains, worse 1-3am and from the cold, thirsty for small amounts of cold water, fear of death, food-poisoning
Bor		Painless diarrhea with mucus	This remedy has an affinity for the nervous system, skin and mucus of the mouth. Thrush, aphthae of mouth, refuse to eat because painful patches inside cheeks, skin looks unhealthy, worse leaning forward/downward/falling motion
Bry		Worse getting up in morning/movement/fruit/hot weather	Very thirsty especially if during a fever, sinuses are very dry (hint to remember: if dry think "bry"), pressure headaches that usually travel from forehead to occiput, or can start from left eye and move to the back of the head
Calc Carb		Diarrhea is sour smelling/watery/with undigested food, worse after drinking milk and teething	Any Calcarea remedy has an affinity for bones, lymph nodes, circulation and polyps. They sweat profusely on head, babies teethe late, walk slow and are lazy, large appetite, remember the four F's: fat, fair skin, fainting, and fearful. If Ruta and Rhus Tox have stopped working, this

		remedy can be thought of. For chronic indications of pulsatilla
Calc Phos	Diarrhea in breast-fed babies	This remedy has an affinity for the bones, blood, lymph nodes and works on the nutrition of the body. Teeth are long, narrow and yellow, bones are long and straight, tired and nervous, rickets, weight loss, repetitive sore throat/bronchitis/colds
Cham	Diarrhea in breast-fed babies/painful/green/hot/smells like rotten eggs, teething	This remedy has an affinity for the digestive system. Hypersensitive to pain, pain feels intolerable, numbness, irritable, angry, moody, hateful, exhausted from teething, insomnia, one cheek is red and hot while other is pale and cold, worse from anger/9pm and 12am/heat(toothache), better from being carried or riding in car
China	Diarrhea is painless and undigested food, indigestion, worse every other day/afternoon/eating/bad meat/after illness/fruit/hot weather/loss of vital fluids/weaning	This remedy is known for ringing and buzzing in ears, hypersensitivity of senses, hypotension, bitter taste in mouth, gas, worse from drafts/slight pressure/every other day/beer/milk/fruit, better from heat and strong pressure, no appetite, loss of vital fluids, pulsating headaches, hemorrhages
Colch	Diarrhea is painful (especially after passing stool)/jelly-like/mucus/watery, worse	This remedy has an affinity for the nervous and digestive system. Acute pain in big toe (gout) that is worse from slightest contact or movement,

	in autumn and getting cold	worse from cold and at night, better from rest and heat, hypersensitive to odors (even food)
Coloc	Diarrhea is green and pasty, colicky, worse after eating/anger/fruit	This remedy has an affinity for the digestive and nervous system. Violent pain causing screaming, cramping pain comes suddenly, worse from anger/rest/left side, better from strong pressure, heat, bending forward, movement, painful diarrhea, facial neuralgia, sciatica
Dulc	Diarrhea is painful and yellow, worse eating cold food/night/damp or cold weather/teething	This remedy has an affinity for respiratory and digestive tract, lymphatic and muscular system, and the skin. Stuffy nose when exposed to cold, wet or rainy weather, catches a cold from air-conditioner, head cold in newborns
Ferr Met	Diarrhea is painless/gassy/undigested food, burping, worse after drinking/while eating/movement/night/teething	This remedy has an affinity for the blood and spleen. Mothers are never the same after childbirth. Pale and blush very easily. Weak, tired, sensitive to cold, cannot make effort, urinate involuntarily when coughing or sneezing or when children play, throbbing headache with hammering pain
Gels	Diarrhea from anticipation anxiety/fright/shock/sad news	This remedy is known for fever (low-grade), circulatory and digestive system, paralysis of nerves and respiratory muscles. Trembling, congestion, sleepy, stiffness, depressed state, worse from heat/hot

		weather/bad news, better from urinating/sweating/movements, thirstless during fever, migraine or congestion headaches, red face
Hep Sul	Painless diarrhea	This remedy is hypersensitive especially to touch and cold air, worse dry/cold weather/slightest draft, better with heat, craves sour things especially vinegar
Ipecac	Diarrhea in infants, grass green color	This remedy has an affinity for the digestive and respiratory system. Hemorrhaging bright red blood, profuse saliva, not thirsty at all, disgusted by food, persistent and violent nausea, vomit is sticky and does not relieve nausea, stools are fermented like yeast, cough with suffocation, large amount of mucus
Mag Carb	Diarrhea is painful/cramping/colicky/frothy/green/slimy/sour-smelling/bitter-smelling, worse before passing stool	This remedy has an affinity for the digestive tract, female genitals, and nervous system. Very sensitive to cold, worse from resting and temperature change, better moving around and walking outside, acute shooting pains along the nerves
Mag Mur	Diarrhea in infants and green color, worse from milk	This remedy has an affinity for the digestive and uterine system. Worse from salt (eating and being by sea) and drinking milk, better by pressure, tongue has teeth marks, constipation with hard stools like that of sheep droppings, migraines better with

		wrapping heat with warm compress
Merc Cor	Diarrhea is painful/burning/severe pain/bloody/green/slimy/smelly/yellow/frequent straining, worse before/during/after passing stool	This remedy has a tendency to produce ulcers very quickly. Any lesion goes from inflammation to ulcers to hemorrhaging. Throat ulcers that burn, burning when urinating
Merc Sol	Diarrhea in infants/painful/burning/bloody/green/slimy/yellow/sweating, worse from cold/evening/night	This remedy has an affinity for the digestive and renal systems with specific action on throat. Foul-smelling breath, gums are white/yellow color and ulcers in gums, tooth abscess, sores in mouth, intense thirst, thick tongue, salivate heavily, parotiditis, heavy perspiration especially at night and offensive in odor, ulcers, worse at night, known as "the human thermometer," shivering and goose-bumps
Nat Mur	Diarrhea in daytime only/painless/gushing/smelly/watery, worse after eating starchy foods, bloating	This remedy can be summed up with three words: Malnutrition, dehydrated and weak. Worse being consoled, worse 10am, worse when at the ocean, loss of vital fluids will cause symptoms, discharge is clear and in large quantities, craves salt, eczema in the creases of joints/forehead/edge of scalp, herpetic rashes especially after illness, dry and cracked skin, chapped lips

Nat Sul	Gurgling and rumbling noises, diarrhea is smelly/thin/gassy (loud and smelly), worse after eating starchy foods/morning/fruit/after getting up in the morning	This remedy has an affinity for digestive, respiratory and nervous system, with effects on the joints and skin, worse from cold and humidity, intense thirst especially for cold drinks, watery stool that squirt out especially in the morning, bronchitis, asthma in children, holds chest when coughing
Nux Vom	Diarrhea is worse after drinking water	This remedy as an affinity for the nervous and digestive system. Irritable, cold, hypersensitive, angry, worse after eating, better with sleep, tongue is yellow/white color, craves spicy and sour food, constipation, sneezing upon waking
Petro	Diarrhea only in daytime/pressing pain/ravenous appetite	This remedy has an affinity for the skin and digestive mucus. Seasickness, worse from cold/winter/motion sickness, better in summer and heat, motion sickness better closing eyes, hands chapped (especially in winter), intense hunger and thirst, diarrhea only in morning
Phos Ac	Diarrhea is profuse/watery/white/without weakness, worse solid food/dry food/summer, rumbling noises	This remedy is severely exhausted especially because of emotional upset. Symptoms are caused by a loss of fluids, indifference to everything, fatigue, painless and orderless diarrhea, urine is milky colored, urine can also be clear in color, hair loss all over body

Phos	Diarrhea is painless/blood-streaked/frequent/profuse/watery/hands and feet are cold, better from cold food, worse from getting chilled	This remedy is highly sensitive especially to light, noises, and smells. Fear of thunderstorm, worse from cold/storms/left side, better from sleep, craves salt and cold drinks, midnight "snacker" especially around 3 am, #1 morning sickness remedy
Podo	Diarrhea alternating with constipation and headache, gurgling and rumbling noises, diarrhea in infants/painless/frequent/gushing/involuntary/profuse/smelly/sudden/exhausting, worse 4am/after drinking water/hot weather/night	This remedy has an affinity for the intestines, liver and female genitals. Worse from hot weather/early in morning/teething, better from lying on abdomen
Puls	Diarrhea in infants/changeable stool/greenish-yellow/slimy/watery, better fresh air, worse after eating/starchy foods/night/rich foods/stuffy room/fruit	This remedy has an affinity for the venous system and mucus. Changeable behavior, worse from heat, better from cold open air, thirstless, thick yellow/yellow-greenish discharge, worse after sunset
Rheum	Diarrhea is pasty and sour smelling, worse from eating unripe fruit	This remedy has an affinity for the liver and intestines. Great teething remedy- restless/temperamental/scalp perspiration, cries when passing stool, sour smell from whole body
Rhus	Diarrhea is mushy and	This remedy has an affinity for the

Tox	watery, worse from getting wet and wet feet	skin, mucus and the nervous system. Better with slow motion and changing of position, shivers when slights part of body is uncovered, perspiration all over body except the face, sprains and dislocations, worse 4-5am and 7pm, intense thirst for cold water or milk
Sil	Gassy (smelly), better with heat/warmth of bed/wrapped up, diarrhea during teething	This remedy has an affinity for the nervous system and is very malnourished. They are weak and demineralized. Worse cold and humid weather, better with heat, slinters (will push them out), fontanels stay open, perspire on head, abscess remedy, white spots on nails, weak nails/hair
Sul	Diarrhea in infants/drives out of bed/burning pain/cramping/painless/slimly/smelly/sour-smelling/watery/gassy (smelly), better from passing gas, worse at 5am/morning/night/standing/beer	This remedy has an affinity for the heart and skin. Worse standing still/heat of bed/water/11am, better perspiring/motion/dry weather, burning sensations all over body, eczema, craves sweets and open air, children look like they have a potbelly, children hate to take baths
Sul Ac	Diarrhea is soft/stringing/yellow, burping, sour vomit	This remedy is for severe weakness. Worse from cold and smell of coffee, better from heat, internal trembling, hemorrhaging black blood
Verat Al	Diarrhea is exhausting/involuntary/burning/cutting/dull/achi	This remedy has an affinity for the digestive and nervous system. Weakness, collapsing, exhaustion,

	ng pain/large amount of diarrhea/green/watery/violent/hands and feet are cold/sweating/vomiting, worse after drinking/movement/getting chilled/fruit	cold sweats on forehead, coldness all over body, burning inside of body, large amounts of vomiting/diarrhea/perspiration, worse cold and humid weather, better heat, cholera-like diarrhea

EARACHE

REMEDIES:

Aconite, Apis, Belladonna, Calcarea Carb., Calcarea Sulph., Chamomilla, Hepar Sulph., Kali Bich., Kali Mur., Kali Sulph., Lachesis, Lycopodium, Magnesia Phos., Mercurius Sol., Nitricum Acidum, Nux Vomica, Pulsatilla, Silica, Sulphur

Remedy	Symptom Differentiation	Keynote Differentiation
Acon	Pain is unbearable, earache from getting chilled and cold-dry wind	This remedy has an affinity for the circulatory and nervous system. Worse extreme or sudden cold/extreme heat/night, better with perspiration, rapid pulse, sudden high fever, red skin, intense thirst for large quantities of cold water, restlessness, anxiety, fear of death, croup cough
Apis	Pain is stinging, earache with sore throat, worse swallowing	This remedy is known for swelling, burning pain, and jealousy. Worse from heat, better from cold, hot dry skin, inflammation

Bell	Pain is spreading down neck/stitching/tearing/throbbing/pain in face, noises in ear, worse on right side	Symptoms usually have sudden and violent onset, local congestion of blood (example face is red), the congested area is usually hot, children usually convulse when they have a fever
Calc Carb	Noises in ear, pain is throbbing	Any Calcarea remedy has an affinity for bones, lymph nodes, circulation and polyps. They sweat profusely on head, babies teethe late, walk slow and are lazy, large appetite, remember the four F's: fat, fair skin, fainting, and fearful. If Ruta and Rhus Tox have stopped working, this remedy can be thought of. For chronic indications of pulsatilla
Calc Sulph	Discharge is blood-streaked/smelly/thick	This remedy has an affinity for the skin and glands. Eczema, pus formations, dizziness, sluggish, eye inflammation, ear discharges pus/blood/thick, croup, gout, worse walking/warm room/milk/movement/bath/night
Cham	Pain is aching/pressing/stitching/unbearable, sensitive to wind, worse bending down and wind	This remedy has an affinity for the digestive system. Hypersensitive to pain, pain feels intolerable, numbness, irritable, angry, moody,

		hateful, exhausted from teething, insomnia, one cheek is red and hot while other is pale and cold, worse from anger/9pm and 12am/heat(toothache), better from being carried or riding in car
Hep Sul	Discharge is smelly, pain is stitching, better wrapped up warmly, worse from cold	This remedy is hypersensitive especially to touch and cold air, worse dry/cold weather/slightest draft, better with heat, craves sour things especially vinegar
Kali Bich	Discharge is smelly/thick/yellow, pain is stitching	This remedy has an affinity for mucus and the skin. Worse cold/2-3am/movement/drinking beer, better with heat, pains start and stop suddenly, aphthae in mouth, thirsty for beer, burning pain in stomach, sciatica left side, heel pain, ulcers, headaches from digestive issues
Kali Mur	Deafness from a cold, swollen glands, noises in ear, worse from swallowing	This remedy has an affinity for the ears and tonsils. Tubal discharge (ears)
Kali Sul	Discharge is thin, ears crackle when chewing	This remedy has an affinity for the mucus and skin. Irritable, angry and obstinate, worse from heat/evening/resting, better

			from cold air/outdoors/walking, throbbing pains, bronchitis, asthma, eczema
	Lach	Earache with sore throat, worse on left side/wind/swallowing	This remedy has an affinity for the nervous system and blood. Bruising, hemorrhaging, blotchy face, talkative, suspicious, jealous, spiteful, depression, worse from discharges that are delayed or insufficient/being touched/sun/heat/sleeping/tight clothes/left side, better from discharge that finally comes out, insomnia (especially before midnight), dreams of ghosts, dead people, coffins, difficulty swallowing, sinusitis, apnea, hot flushes in head, ulcers, bed sores
	Lyc	Pain is tearing, ears feel blocked, noises in ear	This remedy has an affinity for liver and digestion, kidneys and genitals, mucus and skin, and nervous system. Worse between 4-8pm, worse with heat, better with cool air, craving for sweets and oysters, ravenous appetite, flatulence, bloating after meals, doesn't like tight clothes on waist, abdomen is distended, red face after

			eating, migraine from poor digestion, bedwetting, nose stuffy with crusty mucus especially at night, sleep with mouth open, runny nose during day, anorexia in children, fear of new things, "devil at home and angel outside syndrome", lack of self-confidence
	Mag Phos	Spasmodic and shooting pain, better from heat and pressure, worse form cold/turning head/dry wind	This remedy has an affinity for the muscular system. It is a spasmodic remedy. Sudden/intolerable/cramping pains, worse from cold and right side, better from heat and leaning forward
	Merc Sol	Discharge is blood-streaked and smelly, pain is boring/burning/pressing/tearing, ears feel blocked, worse with fresh air/night/warmth of bed	This remedy has an affinity for the digestive and renal systems with specific action on throat. Foul-smelling breath, gums are white/yellow color and ulcers in gums, tooth abscess, sores in mouth, intense thirst, thick tongue, salivate heavily, parotiditis, heavy perspiration especially at night and offensive in odor, ulcers, worse at night, known as "the human thermometer," shivering and goose-bumps
	Nit Ac	Pain is splinter-like and throbbing, ears crackle while	This remedy has an affinity for the body's mucus. Worse

	chewing, sore throat, worse on right side and swallowing	from cold/noise/night, better from heat and riding in the car, prickling pains, craves fatty foods, lips are cracked in corners, anal fissures, plantar warts
Nux Vom	Itching in ear, worse with swallowing, pain is stitching	This remedy as an affinity for the nervous and digestive system. Irritable, cold, hypersensitive, angry, worse after eating, better with sleep, tongue is yellow/white color, craves spicy and sour food, constipation, sneezing upon waking
Puls	Discharge is smelly/thick/yellow-green/yellow, pain is aching/outward/pressing/spreading to neck/stitching/tearing/throbbing, ears feel blocked, noises in ear, deafness, itching in ear, redness of outside of ear, worse at night, earache after measles	This remedy has an affinity for the venous system and mucus. Changeable behavior, worse from heat, better from cold open air, thirstless, thick yellow/yellow-greenish discharge, worse after sunset
Sil	Pain is behind ears and tearing, ears feel blocked, itching in ears	This remedy has an affinity for the nervous system and is very malnourished. They are weak and demineralized. Worse cold and humid weather, better with heat, slinters (will push them out), fontanels stay open, perspire on head, abscess remedy,

			white spots on nails, weak nails/hair
Sul		Pain is aching/lacerating/stitching/tearing, noises in ear, painful, worse on left side and noise	This remedy has an affinity for the heart and skin. Worse standing still/heat of bed/water/11am, better perspiring/motion/dry weather, burning sensations all over body, eczema, craves sweets and open air, children look like they have a potbelly, children hate to take baths

FEVER

Age	Fever	Action
0-2 months	Any temperature above normal	Professional medical advice
2-6 months	>100.5	Professional medical advice
6 + months	>103.5	Professional medical advice after 6 hours of trying remedy
NOTE:	If your child has any of the following symptoms along with the fever, seek IMMEDIATE MEDICAL ADVICE: extreme irritability, stiff neck,	EMERGENCY MEDICAL ATTENTION!

	seizures, vomiting, difficulty breathing	

FEVER/FLU

REMEDIES:

Aconite, Anas Barbariae, Arsenicum Album, Belladonna, Eupatorium, Ferrum Phos., Gelsemium, Influenzinum, Nux Vomica, Pulsatilla, Sulphur

Remedy	Symptom Differentiation	Keynote Differentiation
Acon	Beginning stage of fever, sudden onset, chills (especially when uncovered), thirsty, fever from getting chilled	This remedy has an affinity for the circulatory and nervous system. Worse extreme or sudden cold/extreme heat/night, better with perspiration, rapid pulse, sudden high fever, red skin, intense thirst for large quantities of cold water, restlessness, anxiety, fear of death, croup cough
Anas	First stage of flu, bursting headache, painful cough, flu from cold wind	This remedy is also known as "Oscillococcinum" from the company Boiron and known as the #1 homeopathic flu remedy.
Ars	Very thirsty for sips of water, worse 12-3am (highest fever), chilly, restless	This remedy has an affinity for mucus, kidneys liver, adrenal glands and the nervous system. This remedy can be summed up in three words: weak, restless and cold (temperature-wise). Burning pains, worse 1-3am and from the cold, thirsty for small

		amounts of cold water, fear of death, food-poisoning
Bell	Sudden onset of high fever, face flushed, lips red, hot head, cold hands and feet, delerius	Symptoms usually have sudden and violent onset, local congestion of blood (example face is red), the congested area is usually hot, children usually convulse when they have a fever
Euph	Aching body, bones hurt, chills, worse from 7-9am, soreness in back	This remedy has an affinity for the nose and the eyes. Pink eye, eyes clump together, worse heat/wind/night, better in the dark, measles
Ferr Phos	First stage of fever, slow onset of fever, symptoms like aconite and belladonna but not as intense	Tired, anemic, pale. Bleeds easily, low temperature, rapid pulse, face is red and pale alternatingly, hemorrhages easily, better with slow motion, craves sour things
Gels	Low grade fever, chills, trembling, sleepy, can't open eyes fully, weakness, heaviness, headache, worse from any motion	This remedy is known for fever (low-grade), circulatory and digestive system, paralysis of nerves and respiratory muscles. Trembling, congestion, sleepy, stiffness, depressed state, worse from heat/hot weather/bad news, better from urinating/sweating/movements, thirstless during fever, migraine or congestion headaches, red face

Infl	To prevent flu	Take 2 doses only each in October, January, and March
Nux Vom	Fever from medication side effects, over-eating or loss of sleep, chilliness, worse when uncovered	This remedy as an affinity for the nervous and digestive system. Irritable, cold, hypersensitive, angry, worse after eating, better with sleep, tongue is yellow/white color, craves spicy and sour food, constipation, sneezing upon waking
Puls	Fever with chills, worse in warm room, better in open air and to be uncovered	This remedy has an affinity for the venous system and mucus. Changeable behavior, worse from heat, better from cold open air, thirstless, thick yellow/yellow-greenish discharge, worse after sunset
Sul	Fever with red skin, diarrhea drives out of bed in early morning, thirsty, sweats profusely	This remedy has an affinity for the heart and skin. Worse standing still/heat of bed/water/11am, better perspiring/motion/dry weather, burning sensations all over body, eczema, craves sweets and open air, children look like they have a potbelly, children hate to take baths

HEATSTROKE

ATTENTION! THIS CONSTITUTES A MEDICAL EMERGENCY! Give remedies on the way to the emergency room. Keep child cool.

REMEDIES:

Belladonna, Glonoine

Remedy	Symptom Differentiation	Keynote Differentiation
Bell	Fever, throbbing headache, flushed face, stupor-like, better from bending backward and sitting	Symptoms usually have sudden and violent onset, local congestion of blood (example face is red), the congested area is usually hot, children usually convulse when they have a fever
Glon	Over-exposed to sun, fever with waves of heat, throbbing headache, red face, stupor-like, worse from bending head backward and cold compresses (causes spasms), better from uncovering head and opening eyes	This remedy is known for congestive symptoms. Congestion headaches, surging of blood to head and heart, irregularities in circulation, violent convulsions, worse from exposure to sun/sun rays/gas/open fire/lying down/peaches/6am-12pm/left side

INSOMNIA

REMEDIES:

Aconite, Argentrum Nitricum, Arsenicum Album, Chamomilla, Coffea, Ignatia, Kali Phos., Nux Vomica, Pulsatilla, Rhus Tox., Stramonium, Staphysagria

Remedy	Symptom Differentiation	Keynote Differentiation
Acon	Difficulty falling asleep and staying asleep because fever or anxious dreaming, restless, tossing and turning	This remedy has an affinity for the circulatory and nervous system. Worse extreme or sudden cold/extreme heat/night, better with perspiration, rapid pulse, sudden high fever, red skin, intense thirst for large quantities of cold water, restlessness, anxiety, fear of death, croup cough
Arg Nit	Difficulty falling asleep if room is warm, agitated before bedtime, restless, scary dreams	This remedy has an affinity for the nervous system and the mucus. Nervousness, "what-if," feels as if a thorn is stuck certain part of body, feels like head is expanding, feels squeezing sensation, worse from heat/eating candy/intellectual work/right side, better from fresh air and pressure, vertigo, anticipation anxiety (especially for tests), stomach ulcers

Ars	Restless, anxious, fearful, scary dreams, yelling for help	This remedy has an affinity for mucus, kidneys liver, adrenal glands and the nervous system. This remedy can be summed up in three words: weak, restless and cold (temperature-wise). Burning pains, worse 1-3am and from the cold, thirsty for small amounts of cold water, fear of death, food-poisoning
Cham	Difficulty falling asleep and staying asleep, irritable, pain, refuses things she demanded, sleepy but cannot sleep, better being carried and rocked, moaning, twitching, wants to be uncovered	This remedy has an affinity for the digestive system. Hypersensitive to pain, pain feels intolerable, numbness, irritable, angry, moody, hateful, exhausted from teething, insomnia, one cheek is red and hot while other is pale and cold, worse from anger/9pm and 12am/heat(toothache), better from being carried or riding in car
Coff	Sleepless from hyperactivity, constant ideas, excitable, sensitive to sounds, if breast-feeding mother drinks coffee	This remedy has an affinity for hyperactivity especially of the mind. Intolerance to pain, toothache better from cold water
Ign	Difficulty sleeping because of grief, frequent yawning, very light sleeper,	This remedy is hypersensitive on all organs and senses especially sight and hearing. Very sensitive emotionally

	slightest noise wakes up, jerks, excessive dreaming	especially to sad events, spasms, uncoordinated, sensitive to any sort of excitement or pain, nervous behavior, sighing, fainting, moody, outbreaks of anger, cries easily, irritability, weakness, feels like lump in throat, migraines feel like nails in head, worse 11am/sad news/being consoled/strong smells, better from heat and good time with company, nervous breakdown
Kali Phos	Nightmares, wakes up screaming and cannot go back to sleep, anxious, restless, easily startled	This remedy has an affinity for the nervous and muscular system as well as the blood. Weak, tired, and hypersensitive, worse over-nursing and over-stimulation of mind, discharges are golden, orange or bloody, irritable, moody, headaches in children, nightmares cause insomnia, vaginitis with brown discharge
Nux Vom	Anxiety, dreams of school and fights, sensitive to any noise and irritated by slightest disturbance, wakes at 3-4am, difficulty falling back	This remedy as an affinity for the nervous and digestive system. Irritable, cold, hypersensitive, angry, worse after eating, better with sleep, tongue is yellow/white color, craves spicy and sour food,

		asleep, difficulty sleeping because of side effect of medication	constipation, sneezing upon waking
	Puls	Separation anxiety causes insomnia, repeated thoughts, fear of being alone and dark, nightmares of parents leaving, sleeps with light on, likes to be rocked to sleep, sleeps with hands over head, worse from warm/stuffy room/covered, wakes from being cold	This remedy has an affinity for the venous system and mucus. Changeable behavior, worse from heat, better from cold open air, thirstless, thick yellow/yellow-greenish discharge, worse after sunset
	Rhus Tox	Restlessness, cannot find comfortable position, feels stiff when getting up, better with movement (not initial movement)	This remedy has an affinity for the skin, mucus and the nervous system. Better with slow motion and changing of position, shivers when slights part of body is uncovered, perspiration all over body except the face, sprains and dislocations, worse 4-5am and 7pm, intense thirst for cold water or milk
	Stram	Wakes frequently from nightmares, twitching, convulsions,	This remedy has an affinity for the brain and the nervous system. Worse in dark/shinny and bright objects/being alone, better

		hallucinations	from soft light and being around people, severe and violent convulsions, incoherent talkativeness, hallucinations, nightmares, swollen tongue, doesn't like the sight of liquids, spasmodic and suffocative cough, bright red rash
	Staph	Difficulty falling asleep because of emotional state (thinking of past), abused children, sleepy in the afternoon, frequent yawning and stretching, frightful dreams	This remedy has an affinity for the urinary and genital system as well as the skin. Hypersensitive to emotions, excitable, irritated easily, obsessed about sexual ideas, burning/frequent/dripping urination, eczema with severe itching, styes especially on upper eyelids

Made in the USA
Charleston, SC
02 November 2013